The Washington Manual™ Gastroenterology Subspecialty Consult

Editor
Aaron Shiels, M.D.
Gastroenterology Fellow
Department of Internal Medicine
Division of Gastroenterology
Washington University School of Medicine
Barnes-Jewish Hospital
St. Louis, Missouri

Series Editor
Tammy L. Lin, M.D.
Adjunct Assistant Professor of Medicine
Washington University School of Medicine
St. Louis, Missouri

Series Advisor
Daniel M. Goodenberger, M.D.
Professor of Medicine
Washington University School of Medicine
Chief, Division of Medical Education
Director, Internal Medicine Residency
Program
Barnes-Jewish Hospital
St. Louis, Missouri

 LIPPINCOTT WILLIAMS & WILKINS
A **Wolters Kluwer** Company
Philadelphia · Baltimore · New York · London
Buenos Aires · Hong Kong · Sydney · Tokyo

Acquisitions Editors: Danette Somers and James Ryan
Developmental Editors: Scott Marinaro and Keith Donnellan
Supervising Editors: Allison Risko and Mary Ann McLaughlin
Production Editor: Erica Broennle Nelson, Silverchair Science + Communications
Manufacturing Manager: Colin Warnock
Cover Designer: QT Design
Compositor: Silverchair Science + Communications
Printer: RR Donnelley

©2004 by Department of Medicine, Washington University School of Medicine

Printed in the USA

Library of Congress Cataloging-in-Publication Data

The Washington manual gastroenterology subspecialty consult / [edited by] Aaron Shiels.
   p. ; cm. -- (Washington manual subspecialty consult series)
   Includes bibliographical references and index.
   ISBN 0-7817-4372-9
   1. Gastroenterology--Handbooks, manuals, etc. 2. Digestive
organs--Diseases--Handbooks, manuals, etc. I. Title: Manual gastroenterology
subspecialty consult. II. Shiels, Aaron. III. Series.
   [DNLM: 1. Gastrointestinal Diseases--diagnosis--Handbooks. 2. Gastrointestinal
Diseases--therapy--Handbooks. WI 39 W319 2003]
   RC802.W37 2003
   616.3'3--dc21

                        2003047532

---

10 9 8 7 6 5 4 3 2 1

The Washington Manual™ Gastroenterology Subspecialty Consult

The Washington Manual™ Gastroenterology Subspecialty Consult

Faculty Advisor
Chandra Prakash, M.D.
Assistant Professor
Department of Internal Medicine
Division of Gastroenterology
Washington University School of Medicine
St. Louis, Missouri

Contents

Contributing Authors

John T. Battaile, A.B., M.D.

Clinical Instructor in Medicine
Chief Resident
Department of Internal Medicine
Washington University School of Medicine
St. Louis, Missouri

Ting-hsu Chen, M.D.

Resident Physician
Department of Internal Medicine
Washington University School of Medicine
Barnes-Jewish Hospital
St. Louis, Missouri

Linda A. Cheng, M.D.

Resident Physician
Department of Internal Medicine
Washington University School of Medicine
Barnes-Jewish Hospital
St. Louis, Missouri

Dustin G. James, M.D.

Resident Physician
Department of Internal Medicine
Washington University School of Medicine
Barnes-Jewish Hospital
St. Louis, Missouri

David S. Lotsoff, M.D.

Gastroenterology Fellow
Department of Internal Medicine
Division of Gastroenterology
Washington University School of Medicine
Barnes-Jewish Hospital
St. Louis, Missouri

Patrick B. McDonough, M.D.

Resident Physician
Department of Internal Medicine
Washington University School of Medicine
Barnes-Jewish Hospital
St. Louis, Missouri

Mukul Mehra, M.D.

Gastroenterology Fellow
Department of Internal Medicine
Division of Gastroenterology
Washington University School of Medicine
Barnes-Jewish Hospital
St. Louis, Missouri

Matthew H. Nissing, M.D.

Resident Physician
Department of Internal Medicine
Washington University School of Medicine
Barnes-Jewish Hospital
St. Louis, Missouri

Kevin J. Peifer, M.D.

Gastroenterology Fellow
Department of Internal Medicine
Division of Gastroenterology
Washington University School of Medicine
Barnes-Jewish Hospital
St. Louis, Missouri

Rajesh Shah, M.D.

Resident Physician
Department of Internal Medicine
Washington University School of Medicine
Barnes-Jewish Hospital
St. Louis, Missouri

Varsha V. Shah, M.D.

Resident Physician
Department of Internal Medicine
Washington University School of Medicine
Barnes-Jewish Hospital
St. Louis, Missouri

Aaron Shiels, M.D.

Gastroenterology Fellow
Department of Internal Medicine
Division of Gastroenterology
Washington University School of Medicine
Barnes-Jewish Hospital
St. Louis, Missouri

Clinton T. Snedegar, M.D.

Gastroenterology Fellow
Department of Internal Medicine
Division of Gastroenterology
Washington University School of Medicine
Barnes-Jewish Hospital
St. Louis, Missouri

Sandeep K. Tripathy, M.D., Ph.D.

Gastroenterology Fellow
Department of Internal Medicine
Division of Gastroenterology
Washington University School of Medicine
Barnes-Jewish Hospital
St. Louis, Missouri

Eugene F. Yen, M.D.

Resident Physician
Department of Internal Medicine
Washington University School of Medicine
Barnes-Jewish Hospital
St. Louis, Missouri

Chairman's Note

Medical knowledge is increasing at an exponential rate, and physicians are being bombarded with new facts at a pace that many find overwhelming. The Washington Manual™ Subspecialty Consult Series was developed in this context for interns, residents, medical students, and other practitioners in need of readily accessible practical clinical information. They therefore meet an important unmet need in an era of information overload.

I would like to acknowledge the authors who have contributed to these books. In particular, Tammy L. Lin, M.D., Series Editor, provided energetic and inspired leadership, and Daniel M. Goodenberger, M.D., Series Advisor, Chief of the Division of Medical Education in the Department of Medicine at Washington University, is a continual source of sage advice. The efforts and outstanding skill of the lead authors are evident in the quality of the final product. I am confident that this series will meet its desired goal of providing practical knowledge that can be directly applied to improving patient care.

Kenneth S. Polonsky, M.D.
Adolphus Busch Professor
Chairman, Department of Medicine
Washington University School of Medicine
St. Louis, Missouri

Series Preface

The Washington Manual™ Subspecialty Consult Series is designed to provide quick access to the essential information needed to evaluate a patient on a subspecialty consult service. Each manual includes the most updated and useful information on commonly encountered symptoms or diseases and highlights the practical information you need to gather before formulating a plan. Special efforts have been made to organize the information so that these guides will be valuable and trusted companions for medical students, residents, and fellows. They cover everything from questions to ask during the initial consult to issues in subsequent management.

One of the strengths of this series is that it is written by residents and fellows who know how busy a consult service can be, who know what information will be most helpful, and can detail a practical approach to patient care. Each volume is written to provide enough information for you to evaluate a patient until more in-depth reading can be done on a particular topic. Throughout the series, key references are noted, difficult management situations are addressed, and appropriate practice guidelines are included. Another strength of this series is that it was written in concert. All of the guides were designed to work together.

The most important strength of this series is the collection of authors, faculty advisors, and especially lead authors assembled to write this series. In addition, we received incredible commitment and support from our chairman, Kenneth S. Polonsky, M.D. As a result, the extraordinary depth of talent and genuine interest in teaching others at Washington University is showcased in this series. Although there has always been house staff involvement in editing The Washington Manual™ series, it came to our attention that many of them also wanted to be involved in writing and making decisions about what to convey to fellow colleagues. Remarkably, many of the lead authors became junior subspecialty fellows while writing their guides. Their desire to pass on what they were learning, while trying to balance multiple responsibilities, is a testament to their dedication and skills as clinicians, teachers, and leaders.

We hope this series fulfills the need for essential and practical knowledge for those learning the art of consultation in a particular subspecialty and for those just passing through it.

Tammy L. Lin, M.D., Series Editor
Daniel M. Goodenberger, M.D.,
Series Advisor

Preface

As with many areas of medicine, gastro-enterology is expanding at a rate that can be overwhelming, especially to the physician in training. Even the established practitioner may have difficulty keeping up with changes in disease pathophysiology, diagnostics, and management. To take full advantage of new information, it is essential to have a practical, systematic approach to various gastrointestinal problems. It was with this idea in mind that this handbook was written. Medical students, nurse practitioners, interns, residents, and practicing internists will find this handbook provides an easily accessible reference for handling everyday problems encountered in gastroenterology. Every attempt was made to provide the most relevant information about various gastroenterologic problems.

The handbook is divided into two parts. Part I covers the most common symptoms, signs, or laboratory abnormalities encountered by gastroenterologists. Each chapter is structured in a way that helps the clinician develop a logical, systematic approach to common gastroenterologic problems. Individuals in inpatient consult services as well as outpatient clinics will find this information useful. Presenting symptoms in general gastroenterology, nutrition, and hepatobiliary disease are addressed. In addition to providing a rational approach to these problems, each chapter offers suggested readings for those seeking additional information. Part II addresses the disease states most frequently managed by gastroenterologists. Each chapter is designed to provide key points about the diagnosis and management of these disorders. Again, the objective is to provide the practitioner with an organized approach to each disease entity.

The strength of this handbook lies with the background of the authors. This text was written by gastroenterology fellows and residents who have rotated through the various gastroenterology services at a busy teaching hospital. The authors have experienced first-hand the common questions and problems encountered on the gastroenterology service. This has resulted in the creation of a very practical book that physicians in training and established practitioners will find useful.

I would like to thank Chandra Prakash for his invaluable input as the faculty advisor. I would also like to acknowledge Tammy Lin for the tremendous job she has done as the series editor. She is the common thread that has held this undertaking together, and she has my heartfelt thanks.

A.S.

Key to Abbreviations

AFB	acid-fast bacilli
AFP	α-fetoprotein
AIDS	acquired immunodeficiency syndrome
ALT	alanine transaminase
ANA	antinuclear antibody
aPTT	activated partial thromboplastin time
ARDS	acute respiratory distress syndrome
ASA	aspirin
AST	aspartate transaminase
beta-hCG	beta–human chorionic gonadotrophin
BMI	body mass index
BUN	blood urea nitrogen
CBC	complete blood count
CMV	cytomegalovirus
CNS	central nervous system
COPD	chronic obstructive pulmonary disease
CT	computed tomography
ECG	electrocardiogram
ELISA	enzyme-linked immunosorbent assay
FDA	U.S. Food and Drug Administration
FFP	fresh frozen plasma
GI	gastrointestinal
HBsAg	hepatitis B surface antigen
Hct	hematocrit
HIV	human immunodeficiency virus
HTN	hypertension
ICP	intracranial pressure
ICU	intensive care unit
Ig	immunoglobulin
IM	intramuscular
INR	international normalized ratio
IV	intravenous
NG	nasogastric
NPO	nothing by mouth
NSAIDs	nonsteroidal antiinflammatory drugs
PCR	polymerase chain reaction
PET	positron emission tomography
PID	pelvic inflammatory disease
PO	oral
PT	prothrombin time
RBC	red blood cell
SC	subcutaneous
SGOT	serum glutamic-oxaloacetic transaminase
SGPT	serum glutamic-pyruvic transaminase
SLE	systemic lupus erythematosus

TB	tuberculosis
TMP-SMX	trimethoprim-sulfamethoxazole
TSH	thyroid-stimulating hormone
U/S	ultrasound
VZV	varicella-zoster virus
WBC	white blood cell
WHO	World Health Organization

Introduction to Gastroenterology

Aaron Shiels

Diseases of the digestive tract represent some of the most common and challenging illnesses that health care providers encounter. There is tremendous diversity in the types of digestive diseases that general internists and gastroenterologists manage. Consequently, the field of gastroenterology is broad and offers several subspecialties, including hepatology, pancreatobiliary diseases, and interventional gastroenterology.

Caring for patients presents a challenge to all health care providers, due to both the complexity of the diseases as well as the complex interactions between the brain and the enteric nervous system. Patient experience and expectation modify symptom perception and health care use. Providing good care depends not only on appropriate disease management but also on carefully addressing patient concerns and expectations.

The field of gastroenterology has evolved significantly over the last several decades, primarily due to advances in disease understanding through basic and clinical research. For example, the discovery of *Helicobacter pylori* and the recognition of its key role in peptic ulcer disease have revolutionized the management of gastroduodenal ulcers. Elucidation of the adenoma-carcinoma sequence in colorectal carcinoma has assisted in development of better screening strategies and more effective management of one of the leading causes of cancer mortality. Finally, identification of the hepatitis C virus has revealed a new epidemic that will certainly place a tremendous burden on health care services in the years to come.

Equally important in the evolution of gastroenterology is the development of technology that allows flexible endoscopy to be performed safely and efficiently. Video endoscopy allows direct visualization of much of the GI mucosa. The ability to sample tissue and perform therapeutic intervention has radically changed the approach to acute GI bleeding and GI malignancies. More advanced techniques, such as endoscopic retrograde cholangiopancreatography and endoscopic ultrasonography, now allow accurate diagnosis and treatment of pancreatic and biliary disease and staging of various GI tumors. Newer therapies in the coming years will undoubtedly further advance the ability to manage complex digestive diseases.

The objective of this book is to provide the reader with an easily accessible reference on the common problems faced by a gastroenterologist on a daily basis. An extensive review of each topic is not provided; rather, the information given is practical and applicable to a range of digestive diseases. Key references and articles are provided at the end of each chapter for readers requiring more detailed information.

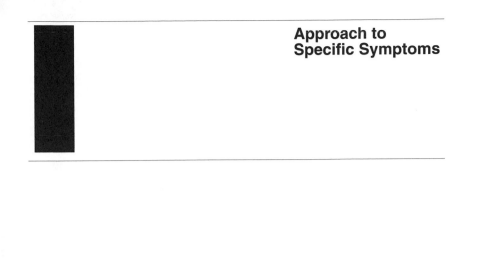

Approach to
Specific Symptoms

2

Dysphagia

Matthew H. Nissing

INTRODUCTION

Dysphagia is defined as difficulty swallowing. It may manifest as a sensation of food "sticking" in the chest or obstruction of passage of food through the oropharynx or esophagus. It must be distinguished from **odynophagia,** which means pain during swallowing. Dysphagia and odynophagia may coexist in the same patient. Globus pharyngeus is the sensation of a lump or fullness in the throat without difficulty swallowing. Finally, some patients may complain of inability to swallow. These patients have aphagia usually caused by food bolus impaction blocking the esophagus.

Classification

Patient history is often very helpful in differentiating between oropharyngeal and esophageal dysphagia. The diagnostic evaluation can then proceed based on the presumed origin of the problem.

- **Oropharyngeal dysphagia** results from defects in the oral and pharyngeal phases of swallowing. These disorders cause problems in preparing the food or transferring it from the oral cavity into the esophagus. Patients report food sticking in their throat, difficulty initiating a swallow, or coughing, choking, drooling, or nasal regurgitation during the swallow.
- **Esophageal dysphagia** results from defects in the esophageal phase of swallowing. Patients describe the sensation of food sticking in the throat or chest, pain in the retrosternal region, or regurgitation some time after swallowing. It is important to try to further delineate whether the esophageal dysphagia is due to a structural or neuromuscular disorder. Structural disorders usually cause dysphagia to solids initially but may later progress to involve liquids as well. Patients with neuromuscular disorders usually report dysphagia for solids and liquids from the beginning.

CAUSES

Pathophysiology

Normal swallowing, one of the most intricate neuromuscular actions in the body, can be divided into three distinct phases: oral, pharyngeal, and esophageal. The oral and pharyngeal phases involve the striated or voluntary muscles of the mouth and pharynx. The initiation is under direct neurologic control. The swallowing control center resides in the medulla and can be activated by either the cerebral cortex (volitional swallowing) or by afferent impulses from the oropharynx (reflexive swallowing).

Oral Phase

The oral phase begins as the food bolus is mechanically prepared by the muscles of the jaw, face, and tongue. It is then propelled posteriorly and superiorly by the tongue and palate. As the bolus passes the anterior tonsillar pillars, the pharyngeal phase begins.

Pharyngeal Phase

The pharyngeal phase continues with the soft palate closing the nasopharynx. The tongue base and pharyngeal constrictors continue to propel the bolus posteriorly. The lips and jaw remain closed, fixing the upper attachments of suprahyoid muscles to allow elevation of the larynx and closure of the laryngeal valves (epiglottis, vocal cords). This enhances airway protection and opens the upper esophageal sphincter (UES). At rest, the UES acts as a barrier against entry of air into the esophagus and regurgitation of material from the esophagus into the pharynx. The entire process takes <1 sec to propel the bolus into the esophagus.

Esophageal Phase

The esophageal phase begins with entry into the esophagus as the UES closes and the bolus is propelled by coordinated muscular contractions. Primary peristalsis in striated muscles is initiated by the act of swallowing via the central program generator in the medulla. Via multiple, complicated control mechanisms, these coordinated contractions are perpetuated through the striated muscle and into the smooth muscle of the more distal esophagus. Secondary peristalsis occurs as a response to distension from retained or refluxed material in the esophagus. The lower esophageal sphincter (LES) is a combination of esophageal smooth muscle and crural diaphragm. The LES relaxes with swallowing/peristaltic contractions via the vagus nerve to allow bolus passage into the stomach.

MANAGEMENT

Diagnostic Evaluation

Oropharyngeal Dysphagia

In most cases, patients have oropharyngeal dysphagia as a manifestation of systemic disorder. Table 2-1 lists the common causes of oropharyngeal dysphagia. The evaluation should begin with a thorough history and physical exam aimed at identifying the underlying cause. Many patients already carry a diagnosis that suggests the underlying disorder. A careful neurologic exam, including direct observation of the patient swallowing water, may also be helpful.

The best initial study for suspected oropharyngeal dysphagia is a **modified barium swallow.** It is a radiographic study in which the oral and pharyngeal phases are observed in real time while the patient swallows barium of various consistencies (thin liquid, thick liquid, barium cookie). This study helps to identify abnormalities of the oropharyngeal phases and may direct therapy, including modification of meal consistency. Patients may tolerate certain consistencies better than others, and the diet can be modified accordingly. If structural lesions are identified, then direct laryngoscopy should be performed. If the modified barium swallow is normal and oropharyngeal dysphagia is still strongly suspected, then the patient should have UES manometry to assess for abnormal UES relaxation.

Esophageal Dysphagia

If esophageal dysphagia is suspected, **barium swallow** or **upper endoscopy** is indicated. Barium swallow is very helpful in the diagnosis of certain motility disorders, including achalasia (classic bird-beak deformity). Barium swallow also commonly reveals structural abnormalities, such as tumors, webs, rings, or strictures. The addition of a solid bolus (barium marshmallow or pill) aids in the detection of subtle abnormalities. Upper endoscopy is useful as the initial test in evaluating esophageal dysphagia, or it may be used to evaluate an abnormal barium swallow. Endoscopy allows direct visualization of the esophagus and permits tissue biopsy of structural lesions. If endoscopy and barium swallow are normal, or if a motility disorder is suspected, then motility studies of the esophagus and LES should be performed. The diagnosis of achalasia is best made with motility studies. Other primary and secondary motor disorders can also be diagnosed using motility studies. Table 2-2 lists the common causes of esophageal dysphagia.

TABLE 2-1. CAUSES OF OROPHARYNGEAL DYSPHAGIA

Neuromuscular disorders
  Cerebrovascular accident
  Parkinson's disease
  Amyotrophic lateral sclerosis
  Poliomyelitis
  Polymyositis
  Myasthenia gravis
  Brain tumors
  Hypothyroidism
  Abnormal upper esophageal sphincter relaxation
Structural lesions
  Neoplasm
  Inflammation (pharyngitis, radiation)
  Plummer-Vinson syndrome
  Cervical hyperostosis
  Thyromegaly
  Lymphadenopathy
  Prior oropharyngeal surgery
  Zenker's diverticulum

Treatment

Oropharyngeal Dysphagia

Therapy is directed at the underlying disorder, if possible. Many patients have irreversible or progressive neurologic diseases that lead to worsening oropharyngeal dys-

TABLE 2-2. CAUSES OF ESOPHAGEAL DYSPHAGIA

Structural causes
  Benign stricture
  Esophageal cancer
  Schatzki's ring
  Esophageal webs
  Foreign bodies
  Extrinsic (vascular, cervical osteoarthritis, adenopathy)
Motility disorders
  Achalasia
  Scleroderma
  Hypertensive lower esophageal sphincter
  Diffuse esophageal spasm
  Chagas' disease
  Nutcracker esophagus

phagia. Consultation with a speech therapist is often helpful to provide modifications in eating behaviors and food consistency. Even with these interventions, many patients have such severe oropharyngeal dysphagia that continued oral intake places them at excessive risk of aspiration or inadequate caloric intake. If the prognosis warrants, consideration for alternative means of feeding should be pursued, including placement of percutaneous or surgical gastrostomy tubes.

Esophageal Dysphagia

As with oropharyngeal causes, management should be tailored to the underlying disorder. See Chap. 14, Esophageal Disorders, for a discussion of the specific management of the common esophageal disorders. Endoscopic therapy is available for many of the structural causes of esophageal dysphagia, including dilation of strictures and disruption of esophageal rings. Obstructing tumors may be treated with dilation or by endoscopic stenting. Some motility disorders are also amenable to endoscopic therapy, including botulinum toxin injections of the LES for patients with achalasia. Percutaneous or surgical gastrostomy tube placement is often required for patients with tumors that cannot be dilated or stented.

KEY POINTS TO REMEMBER

- Dysphagia, or difficulty swallowing, must be differentiated from odynophagia, which is painful swallowing.
- Oropharyngeal dysphagia results from defects in the oral and pharyngeal phases of swallowing. Patients experience food sticking in their throat, difficulty initiating a swallow, or coughing, choking, drooling, or nasal regurgitation during the swallow.
- Esophageal dysphagia results from defects in the esophageal phase of swallowing. Patients describe the sensation of food sticking in the throat or chest, pain in the retrosternal region, or regurgitation some time after swallowing.
- Structural disorders usually cause dysphagia to solids initially but may later progress to involve liquids as well. Patients with neuromuscular disorders usually report dysphagia for solids and liquids from the beginning.
- The best initial study for suspected oropharyngeal dysphagia is a modified barium swallow.
- Upper endoscopy is useful as the initial test in evaluating esophageal dysphagia, or it may be used to evaluate an abnormal barium swallow.

REFERENCES AND SUGGESTED READINGS

Clouse RE. Functional esophageal disorders. *Gut* 1999;45SII:II31–II36.

Cook IJ, Kahrilas PJ. AGA technical review on management of oropharyngeal dysphagia. *Gastroenterology* 1999;116(2):455–478.

Schechter GL. Systemic causes of dysphagia in adults. *Otolaryngol Clin North Am* 1998;31(3):525–535.

Shapiro J. Evaluation and treatment of swallowing disorders. *Compr Ther* 2000;26 (3):203–209.

Spechler SJ. AGA technical review on treatment of patients with dysphagia caused by benign disorders of the distal esophagus. *Gastroenterology* 1999;117(1):233–254.

Spieker MR. Evaluating dysphagia. *Am Fam Physician* 2000;61(12):3639–3648.

Nausea and Vomiting

Rajesh Shah

INTRODUCTION

Nausea refers to the feeling of an imminent urge to vomit and is usually sensed in the throat or epigastrium. **Vomiting** (or emesis), in turn, denotes the forceful ejection of upper GI contents through the mouth. It is important to distinguish these symptoms from regurgitation and rumination. **Regurgitation** is the passive retrograde flow of esophageal contents into the mouth, commonly seen in gastroesophageal reflux. **Rumination** is the effortless regurgitation of recently ingested food into the mouth, followed by rechewing and swallowing. These two conditions have very different etiologies and therapy.

Nausea may precede the act of emesis, occur concurrently, or occur on its own. Generally, altered autonomic activity and decreased function of the upper GI tract accompany severe nausea. The act of emesis is a highly coordinated event requiring the integration of both the central and peripheral nervous system.

Nausea and vomiting (N/V) contribute significantly to increased hospital costs and physician visits and also frequently prompt consultation with a gastroenterologist. It is important to note, however, that although GI causes of N/V are common, there are a number of systemic, neurologic, and metabolic disorders that frequently contribute as well.

CAUSES

Pathophysiology

Initiation of Emesis

The vomiting center, located in the dorsal portion of the lateral reticular formation, serves as the point of integration and initiation of emesis. Afferent stimuli are received by the vomiting center from a variety of sources. The vestibular system, particularly the labyrinthine apparatus located in the inner ear, sends afferent signals through the vestibular nucleus and the cerebellum to the vomiting center. Peripheral neural pathways from the GI tract play a large role in the initiation of emesis. Afferent vagal fibers project to the nucleus tractus solitarius and from there to the vomiting center. Serotonergic pathways are also believed to play a large role in peripheral stimulation via 5-hydroxytryptamine-3 (5-HT_3) receptors located on the afferent vagal nerves. The chemoreceptor trigger zone, located in the area postrema on the floor of the fourth ventricle, is a major mediator of the initiation of emesis. A number of drugs and toxins activate the zone via dopamine D_2, muscarinic M_1, histaminergic H_1, serotonergic 5-HT_3, and vasopressinergic receptors. A number of metabolic abnormalities also affect the trigger zone. Once activated, efferent signals are sent on to the vomiting center, where the physical act of emesis is initiated.

Mechanism of Emesis

Efferent pathways from the vomiting center serve to initiate the mechanism of vomiting. Important pathways include the phrenic nerves to the diaphragm, the spinal nerves to the abdominal musculature, and visceral efferent vagal fibers to the larynx, pharynx, esophagus, and stomach.

The act of emesis involves a coordinated sequence of events involving the abdominal wall musculature as well as the muscular walls of the GI tract. While the gastroesophageal sphincter and the gastric body relax, a combination of forceful contractions of the abdominal wall muscles, diaphragm, and gastric pylorus causes the expulsion of gastric contents into the esophagus. Reverse peristalsis of the esophagus propels these contents into mouth, while reflex closure of the glottis prevents aspiration and elevation of the soft palate prevents reflux into the nasopharynx.

Differential Diagnosis

A broad array of disease processes can produce N/V. Table 3-1 lists some of the common causes.

TABLE 3-1. COMMON CAUSES OF NAUSEA AND VOMITING

Medications
  Chemotherapy: cisplatinum, dacarbazine, nitrogen mustard
  Analgesics
  Oral contraceptives
  Digoxin
  Antiarrhythmics
  Beta blockers
  Antibiotics: erythromycin, tetracycline, sulfonamides
  Sulfasalazine
  Azathioprine
  Antiparkinsonian medications
  Theophylline
  Narcotics
Infections
  Gastroenteritis
    Viral: rotavirus, Norwalk virus, adenovirus, reovirus
  Bacterial: *Staphylococcus aureus*, *Salmonella*, *Bacillus cereus*, and *Clostridium perfringens* (toxins)
  Non-GI infections
GI and peritoneal disorders
  Peptic ulcer disease
  Appendicitis
  Hepatitis
  Mesenteric ischemia
  Cholecystitis
  Gastric outlet obstruction
  Small bowel obstruction
  Gastroparesis
  Nonulcer dyspepsia
CNS disorders
  Increased intracranial pressure: tumor, hemorrhage, pseudotumor cerebri

(continued)

TABLE 3-1. CONTINUED

Migraine
Psychogenic vomiting
Cyclic vomiting syndrome
Anorexia nervosa
Bulimia nervosa
Labyrinthine disorders
Other disorders
Pregnancy
Uremia
Diabetic ketoacidosis
Addison's disease
Postop nausea and vomiting
Cardiac ischemia/infarction

Medications

Antiparkinsonian agents (e.g., L-dopa, bromocriptine), nicotine, digoxin, and opiate analgesics produce N/V through direct action on receptors in the chemoreceptor trigger zone. NSAIDs and antibiotics, such as erythromycin, stimulate peripheral afferent pathways to activate the vomiting center directly. Chemotherapeutic agents frequently cause N/V through several mechanisms. Acute vomiting, usually caused by agents such as cisplatinum, nitrogen mustard, and dacarbazine, is generally mediated through serotonergic pathways, both centrally and peripherally. Delayed and anticipatory vomiting are serotonin independent.

Infections

Viral gastroenteritis is a common cause of acute N/V, particularly in the pediatric population. Causative agents include rotavirus, Norwalk virus, reovirus, and adenovirus. Bacterial infections with *Staphylococcus aureus*, *Salmonella*, *Bacillus cereus*, and *Clostridium perfringens* are commonly associated with "food poisoning." Enterotoxins act both centrally and peripherally. Miscellaneous infectious processes, such as otitis media, meningitis, and acute hepatitis, also commonly produce N/V.

GI and Peritoneal Disorders

Functional disorders of motility constitute a large percentage of cases of chronic N/V. Alterations in motility are present but correlate poorly with symptoms. Gastroparesis is associated with a multitude of systemic disorders, notably diabetes mellitus, SLE, scleroderma, and amyloidosis. Intestinal or gastric outlet obstruction often causes nausea that is relieved with vomiting. Dyspepsia is often related to gastroesophageal reflux disease or peptic ulcer disease but is also frequently functional in nature.

Inflammation of any viscus can cause N/V through activation of afferent pathways. Pancreatitis, appendicitis, cholecystitis, and biliary pain (colic) are common causes. Peritoneal inflammation is usually associated with severe abdominal pain.

CNS Disorders

Increased intracranial pressure due to any cause (malignancy, infection, cerebrovascular accident, hemorrhage) can induce emesis with or without nausea. Labyrinthine disorders, including labyrinthitis, tumors, Ménière's disease, and motion sickness, are common causes of N/V.

Endocrine and Metabolic Disorders

Uremia, diabetic ketoacidosis, and hypercalcemia are postulated to cause N/V through direct action on the area postrema. Parathyroid, thyroid, and adrenal disease act by disruption of GI motility. The nausea of pregnancy deserves special mention. It occurs in approximately 70% of women during the first trimester. The symptoms typically peak around the ninth week and subside by the end of the first trimester. The cause of nausea in pregnancy is likely related to fluctuations in hormones, as the symptoms parallel the rise and fall of beta–hCG levels. Hyperemesis gravidarum complicates 1–5% of pregnancies, causing intractable vomiting. This condition is serious and can result in inability to gain weight or significant weight loss.

PRESENTATION

History

Acute vomiting suggests infection, medication or toxin induced, or accumulation of toxins as in uremia or diabetic ketoacidosis. Chronic vomiting, defined as emesis for ≥ 1 mo, suggests a chronic medical or psychiatric condition.

Timing of vomiting can also suggest an etiology. Vomiting that occurs within minutes of a meal can be caused by an obstructive process in the proximal GI tract. Inflammatory conditions generally produce vomiting approximately 1 hr after meals, whereas vomiting from gastroparesis can occur several hours later. Early morning vomiting often occurs with first-trimester pregnancy and uremia.

Vomiting of undigested foods may suggest an esophageal process such as achalasia, whereas vomiting of partially digested foods suggests gastric retention due to obstruction or gastroparesis. Blood or the appearance of "coffee grounds" in the emesis indicates an upper GI bleed. Bile rules out the possibility of obstruction proximal to the duodenal papilla. Foul odor can indicate a more distal obstruction, fistula, or bacterial overgrowth.

Abdominal pain is commonly associated with N/V and may indicate an inflammatory condition, such as appendicitis or pancreatitis. Diarrhea or fever suggests an infectious process. Weight loss occurs with chronic vomiting. Mental status changes and headache may indicate meningitis or other CNS pathology. Vertigo and tinnitus suggest a labyrinthine process.

Physical Exam

Assessment of volume status should be the initial focus of the physical exam. Orthostatic hypotension and tachycardia indicate hypovolemia and should be corrected immediately with volume resuscitation. Exam of the oropharynx may reveal loss of dental enamel, often found in bulimia. Abdominal tenderness suggests an inflammatory condition, and rebound tenderness suggests peritonitis. Absence of bowel sounds is consistent with intestinal ileus, whereas obstruction classically presents with high-pitched, hyperactive bowel sounds. Hepatomegaly or a tender liver edge may indicate hepatitis. Neurologic exam can reveal signs of meningitis and other CNS disorders.

MANAGEMENT

Diagnostic Evaluation

Lab tests should include a basic metabolic panel. Hyponatremia and elevated BUN and creatinine are seen with dehydration. Hypokalemia and contraction alkalosis are also seen with prolonged vomiting and dehydration and result from a hyperaldosterone state. Liver chemistries may reveal acute hepatitis or cholestasis. Elevated lipase and amylase indicate pancreatitis. A CBC is useful to rule out blood loss with decreased hemoglobin and Hct. An elevated WBC count suggests an infectious process. Of note, it is important to exclude pregnancy in women of reproductive age with acute vomiting by checking urine or serum beta–hCG levels.

Diagnostic Procedures

Initial diagnostic testing should include radiographic evaluation with flat and upright plain films of the abdomen. The presence of air-fluid levels and small bowel dilatation demonstrates obstruction. Free air under the diaphragm indicates bowel perforation. Small bowel follow through with barium contrast can further evaluate for subtle obstruction and mucosal lesions. CT of the abdomen may be useful in evaluating the liver, pancreas, and biliary system, as well as small and large intestines. Esophagogastroduodenoscopy and colonoscopy allow direct visualization of GI mucosa. Further diagnostic studies include gastric emptying scans, GI manometry, and electrogastrography.

Treatment

Orthostatic hypotension and sinus tachycardia are signs of hypovolemia (with loss of approximately 10% of circulating blood volume) and should be corrected immediately with administration of IV fluids. Patients with severe comorbid conditions should be hospitalized, as dehydration may be more severe.

Medical Therapy

Therapy should be directed at the specific etiology of N/V. Emesis due to peptic ulcer disease can be treated by acid suppression and eradication of *Helicobacter pylori*. Many inflammatory conditions, such as appendicitis and cholecystitis, as well as small bowel or gastric outlet obstruction, require surgical intervention. Antiemetic and promotility agents are useful for symptomatic relief. Patients with chronic functional vomiting syndromes may benefit from low-dose anticholinergics. It is important to note that many patients with acute, self-limited N/V may only require observation, antiemetics, and hydration.

Antiemetic Medications

- Antihistamines can be useful for symptomatic relief. Meclizine (25 mg PO qid) is used for labyrinthitis, whereas promethazine (12.5–25 mg PO/IM/IV q6h) is very useful in treating the nausea caused by uremia.
- Anticholinergics, such as scopolamine (1.5-mg patch q 3 days), are used for the nausea of motion sickness. Scopolamine may be prescribed in the form of a transdermal patch.
- Dopamine receptor antagonists [prochlorperazine (5–10 mg PO/IM/IV q6h), chlorpromazine (10–50 mg PO/IM q8h)] are commonly used for both chronic and acute vomiting. Side effects are due to action on dopamine receptors throughout the CNS and include drowsiness, insomnia, anxiety, mood changes, confusion, dystonic reactions, tardive dyskinesia, and parkinsonian symptoms.
- 5-HT$_3$ receptor antagonists [ondansetron (4–8 mg PO/IV q8h), granisetron (1 mg PO q12h)] are very useful in nausea caused by chemotherapeutic agents, particularly cisplatin. Corticosteroids and cannabinoids also exert potent antiemetic effects in patients undergoing chemotherapy.

Prokinetic Agents

- Metoclopramide (5–20 mg PO qid) acts on 5-HT$_4$ receptors and peripheral dopamine receptors and is used for gastroparesis and chemotherapy-induced nausea.
- Cisapride is no longer available in the United States due to its proarrhythmic effects.
- Domperidone, also a peripheral dopamine receptor antagonist, is a potent prokinetic agent but is not currently available in the United States.

Other Agents

Low-dose TCAs (amitriptyline or nortriptyline, 10–50 mg PO qhs) are useful in functional vomiting syndromes.

KEY POINTS TO REMEMBER

• The chemoreceptor trigger zone, located in the area postrema on the floor of the fourth ventricle, is a major mediator of the initiation of emesis.

• Viral gastroenteritis is a common cause of acute N/V, particularly in the pediatric population.

• Functional disorders constitute a large percentage of cases of chronic N/V.

• Acute vomiting suggests infection, medication or toxin induced, or accumulation of toxins as in uremia or diabetic ketoacidosis. Chronic vomiting, occurring for ≥ 1 mo, suggests a chronic medical or psychiatric condition.

• Orthostatic hypotension and tachycardia indicate hypovolemia and should be corrected immediately with volume resuscitation.

• Dopamine receptor antagonists (prochlorperazine, chlorpromazine) are commonly used for both chronic and acute vomiting.

REFERENCES AND SUGGESTED READINGS

Prakash C, Lustman PJ, Freedland KE, et al. Tricyclic antidepressants for functional nausea and vomiting: clinical outcome in 37 patients. *Dig Dis Sci* 1998;43:1951–1956.

Quigley EMM. Gastric and small intestinal motility in health and disease. *Gastroenterol Clin North Am* 1996;25:113–145.

Quigley EMM, Hasler WL, Parkman HP. AGA technical review on nausea and vomiting. *Gastroenterology* 2001;120:263–286.

Talley NJ, Phillips SF. Non-ulcer dyspepsia: potential causes and pathophysiology. *Ann Intern Med* 1988;108:865–879.

Talley NJ, Silverstein MD, Agreus L, et al. AGA technical review: evaluation of dyspepsia. *Gastroenterology* 1998;114:582–595.

Watcha MF, White PF. Postoperative nausea and vomiting: its etiology, treatment and prevention. *Anesthesiology* 1993;78:403–406.

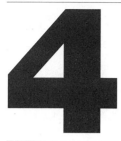

Diarrhea

Kevin J. Peifer

INTRODUCTION

Definition

The best working definition of **diarrhea** is an increased liquidity or decreased consistency of stools. Many experts consider increased frequency of bowel movements, specifically >3 stools/day, as part of this definition. In the past, *diarrhea* was defined medically as a stool weight of more than 200–300 g/24 hrs. However, some people have increased fecal weight with normal stool consistency, whereas others have normal stool weights with increased liquidity and stool frequency. In the normal state, nearly 10 L of fluid enter the jejunum on a daily basis. This volume is reduced to 1 L on entering the colon. Absorption in the colon further reduces the fluid volume lost in stool to only 100 mL/day. Thus, in the normal state, the intestine is highly efficient in its reabsorption of water.

Classification

Diarrhea is generally caused by changes in water and electrolyte transport. These changes can occur as a result of impaired absorption, increased secretion, or both. There are four general mechanisms by which diarrhea occurs.

Osmotic Diarrhea

Osmotic diarrhea results from large amounts of poorly absorbable, osmotically active solutes in the intestinal tract. Osmotic diarrhea has two clinical hallmarks that help lead to its diagnosis. First, the diarrhea ceases with fasting; second, the stool osmotic gap is abnormally elevated. The stool osmotic gap can be determined by measuring the stool $[Na^+]$ and $[K^+]$ and calculating as follows:

$$\text{Stool osmotic gap} = 290 - 2\,(Na^+ + K^+)$$

The osmotic gap is normally <50 mOsm/kg. In pure osmotic diarrhea, the osmotic gap is usually >125 mOsm/kg. Under normal circumstances, as stool passes from the rectum, fecal osmolality is equal to serum osmolality, which is approximately 290 mOsm/kg. The most common causes of osmotic diarrhea are disaccharidase deficiencies, which lead to carbohydrate malabsorption. Of these deficiencies, lactase deficiency is the most prevalent. Nearly three-fourths of nonwhites and one-fourth of whites have lactase deficiency.

Secretory Diarrhea

Secretory diarrhea is caused by increased intestinal secretion or decreased absorption. This results in large amounts of watery diarrhea (1–10 L/24 hrs), and the diarrhea is typically painless. In this type of diarrhea, the stool osmotic gap is normal, and the diarrhea usually persists during fasting, although at times at a reduced rate. Some of the common causes of secretory diarrhea are endocrine tumors, bile salt malabsorption, and laxative abuse. The prototypical secretory diarrhea occurs in cholera in which the cholera toxin stimulates large amounts of sodium and chloride excretion in intestinal crypt cells, with resultant profuse watery diarrhea.

Inflammatory Diarrhea
Diarrhea in inflammatory disorders results from disruption of the integrity of the intestinal mucosa. Inflammation and ulceration lead to discharge of mucus, serum protein, and blood into the bowel lumen. Infectious colitis and inflammatory bowel disease (IBD) are common causes of this type of diarrhea.

Motility Disorders
Diarrhea may be associated with abnormal bowel motility secondary to systemic disorders or surgery. Irritable bowel syndrome is the most common condition in this category. Carcinoid syndrome, hyperthyroidism, and some medications, such as prostaglandins, may produce diarrhea by causing abnormally increased bowel motility. Intestinal dysmotility or pancreatic exocrine insufficiency may cause diarrhea secondary to bacterial overgrowth. Visceral neuromyopathies may cause diarrhea as well. The most notable is diabetic diarrhea, which usually occurs concomitantly with autonomic and peripheral neuropathies.

ACUTE DIARRHEA

Acute diarrhea is defined as diarrhea persisting <*4 wks*. Worldwide, more than 2 billion people experience ≥ 1 episode of acute diarrhea each year. As a result of poor sanitation and limited access to health care, acute infectious diarrhea remains one of the most common causes of death in developing countries. In these countries, infectious diarrhea often adversely affects children, accounting for >5 million deaths/yr. In the United States, nearly 100 million people are affected by acute diarrhea annually. Nearly half of these individuals must limit their activities, 250,000 require hospitalization, and approximately 3000 people die. Most deaths occur in the debilitated and the elderly. Most cases of acute diarrhea are mild and are caused by self-limited processes, lasting <5 days. Nearly 90% of cases require no diagnostic evaluation and respond to simple rehydration therapy.

Causes

Differential Diagnosis
The most common causes of acute diarrhea are infectious agents, bacterial toxins, and drugs. Table 4-1 lists the most common causes of infectious diarrhea. Less common causes include IBD, radiation colitis, ischemic colitis, fecal impaction, ingestion of poorly absorbable sugars, and pelvic inflammation.

TABLE 4-1. CAUSES OF ACUTE INFECTIOUS DIARRHEA

Viruses	*Clostridium difficile*
Adenovirus	*Escherichia coli* O157:H7
Norwalk virus	Enterotoxigenic *E. coli*
Rotavirus	*Yersinia*
Bacteria	Parasites
Campylobacter	*Entamoeba histolytica*
Salmonella	*Giardia lamblia*
Shigella	*Cyclospora*

Presentation

History
A detailed history helps narrow the differential diagnosis and, when combined with the physical exam, dictates whether a diagnostic workup needs to be performed. The character and duration of diarrhea are important as well as a detailed medication history, including laxatives, antibiotics, and over-the-counter medications. Recent travel to endemic areas may suggest traveler's diarrhea or parasite infection. A history of recent immigration from a developing country or immunosuppression should place parasite infection higher on the differential.

Persons with noninflammatory diarrhea often have watery, nonbloody diarrhea associated with periumbilical cramps, bloating, nausea, or vomiting. This type of diarrhea is usually caused by disruption of normal absorption and secretory processes in the small intestine. In most cases, the diarrhea is mild. However, it may become voluminous, ranging from 10–200 mL/kg/24 hrs, which can result in dehydration and electrolyte abnormalities.

Inflammatory diarrhea often presents with fever and bloody diarrhea. These infections predominantly involve the colon, with small-volume diarrhea defined as <1 L/day. Abdominal pain and tenesmus are usually present as well. Because these infectious agents are often invasive, fecal leukocytes are usually present. IBD may present acutely with fever, abdominal pain, and bloody diarrhea, which can make it indistinguishable from infectious diarrhea.

Physical Exam
A complete physical exam should be performed, paying particular attention to volume status and signs of severe abdominal tenderness or peritonitis. Hospitalization is necessary in cases of severe dehydration, toxicity, or marked abdominal pain.

Management

Diagnostic Evaluation
Most cases of acute diarrhea are mild and self-limited. However, several clinical findings necessitate immediate evaluation and diagnostic testing. For example, patients with signs of inflammatory diarrhea with high fever (>38.5°C), bloody diarrhea, or abdominal pain should be promptly evaluated. Patients with orthostatic hypotension, presyncope, excess thirst, dry mouth, oliguria, or profuse watery diarrhea should receive aggressive volume resuscitation. Frail, elderly individuals and immunocompromised patients should also be evaluated urgently.

Stool bacterial cultures have a sensitivity of only 40–60%, although this can be improved by sending at least three samples. Patients with a history of recent antibiotic use should have their stool analyzed for *Clostridium difficile* toxin. Any patient whose diarrhea persists >10 days should have three stool samples sent for ova and parasites. Further, sigmoidoscopy may be warranted in cases of severe proctitis or suspected *C. difficile* colitis. Often, sigmoidoscopy is helpful in distinguishing infectious diarrhea from ischemic colitis or IBD. A stool wet mount exam should be considered in sexually active male homosexuals to look for amebiasis. In addition, any sexually active patient in whom acute proctitis is suspected should have a rectal swab cultured to rule out chlamydia, *Neisseria gonorrhea*, and herpes simplex virus.

Treatment
Patients with uncomplicated, mild, acute diarrhea are treated with oral fluids containing carbohydrates and electrolytes. These patients may find further comfort with bowel rest, which includes avoiding high-fiber foods, fats, milk products, caffeine, and alcohol. In more severe diarrhea, volume depletion occurs, which may necessitate IV fluids. Lactated ringers or 0.9% normal saline should be given in these cases at a rate of 50–200 mL/kg/24 hrs, depending on the severity of the hypovolemia.

In cases of mild to moderate diarrhea, antidiarrheal agents are safe and may improve patient comfort. Patients with bloody diarrhea, high fever, or systemic toxicity should not be given antidiarrheals. Anticholinergic agents are absolutely contraindicated in acute diarrhea due to the rare complication of toxic megacolon. If the decision to use an antidiarrheal agent is made, in most cases, loperamide is the agent of choice. Initially, 4 mg of loperamide is given PO followed by 2 mg after each loose stool up to a maximum daily dose of 16 mg. In patients with suspected traveler's diarrhea, 30 mL of bismuth subsalicylate given qid may reduce symptoms through its antiinflammatory and antibacterial properties.

Empiric treatment with antibiotics is only recommended in cases of suspected invasive bacterial infection, which is suggested by high fever, tenesmus, bloody diarrhea, or fecal leukocytes. The drug of choice is a fluoroquinolone for 5–7 days. Alternative antibiotics are TMP-SMX or erythromycin. If *Giardia* is suspected, metronidazole may be given. Antibiotic treatment is also recommended in infectious diarrhea caused by amebiasis, cholera, *C. difficile*, *Shigella*, extraintestinal *Salmonella*, traveler's diarrhea, and STDs (chlamydia, gonorrhea, herpes simplex virus, and syphilis). In general, antibiotics are not recommended for patients with nontyphoid *Salmonella*, *Campylobacter*, *Aeromonas*, *Yersinia*, or *Escherichia coli* O157:H7 except in severe cases, as antibiotics have not been shown to hasten recovery or decrease the contagious period in these bacterial infections.

CHRONIC DIARRHEA

Chronic diarrhea persists ≥ *4 wks* and usually requires diagnostic evaluation. In contrast to acute diarrhea, chronic diarrhea often has a noninfectious etiology. Chronic diarrhea has an estimated prevalence of 3–5%. There are numerous causes, but a careful and detailed history and physical exam along with selective testing often yield an accurate diagnosis.

Causes

Differential Diagnosis
Table 4-2 lists the classes and most common causes of chronic diarrhea. The most common cause is irritable bowel syndrome. Other common causes include lactose intolerance (lactase deficiency), IBD, and bowel impaction.

TABLE 4-2. CLASSIFICATION OF CHRONIC DIARRHEA

Secretory diarrhea	Steatorrhea
Carcinoid syndrome	Pancreatic insufficiency
Vasoactive intestinal polypeptide tumor	Bacterial overgrowth
Zollinger-Ellison syndrome	Celiac sprue
Medullary thyroid carcinoma	Whipple's disease
Villous adenoma	Short bowel syndrome
Microscopic colitis	Abetalipoproteinemia
Inflammatory diarrhea	Altered intestinal motility
Inflammatory bowel disease	Irritable bowel syndrome
Infectious colitis	Hyperthyroidism
Radiation enterocolitis	Diabetes mellitus
Eosinophilic enterocolitis	Fecal impaction
Osmotic diarrhea	
Lactase deficiency	
Laxative abuse	

Presentation

History and Physical Exam

As in acute diarrhea, a comprehensive history is important to help direct the diagnostic workup. It is important to elicit the onset, duration, pattern, aggravating factors (paying special attention to diet and medications), and relieving factors as well as characteristics of the patient's stool. It is important to distinguish whether the stools are watery, bloody, or fatty. In addition, patients should be questioned about fever, pain, presence or absence of fecal incontinence, and weight loss. A history of diabetes, thyroid problems, or other autoimmune disorders may be pertinent. Often, IBD is preceded by years of seronegative spondyloarthropathy. A complete surgical history may also give clues to the etiology, in particular gastric surgery, bowel resections, or cholecystectomy. In most cases of chronic diarrhea, the physical exam is less revealing than the patient's history but should focus on volume status and evidence of malnutrition.

Management

Diagnostic Evaluation

A CBC may reveal anemia suggesting blood loss or malnutrition. Leukocytosis favors an inflammatory cause, whereas eosinophilia may suggest parasite infection or eosinophilic gastroenteritis. Serum chemistry screening may identify coexistent liver disease and electrolyte abnormalities. Tests of thyroid function should be performed to evaluate for hyperthyroidism.

Before pursuing an extensive evaluation, it is often appropriate at this point to initiate a therapeutic trial if a specific diagnosis is suspected. If the patient's diarrhea resolves with empiric treatment, the diagnosis is essentially confirmed and no further workup is necessary. However, if symptoms persist, further studies should be performed. In nearly two-thirds of cases, the etiology of a patient's chronic diarrhea remains unclear after the initial history, physical exam, and basic lab work have been completed.

Stool Studies

Quantitative stool analysis often provides information about the severity and type of diarrhea, helping to guide further investigations. The following studies may be useful:

- **Stool osmotic gap:** Using the formula listed above, the osmotic gap can be calculated. Secretory diarrheas typically have osmotic gaps <50 mOsm/kg, whereas osmotic diarrheas have osmotic gaps >125 mOsm/kg.
- **Stool pH:** pH <5.6 suggests carbohydrate malabsorption.
- **Fecal occult blood testing:** The presence of occult blood suggests mucosal damage, including IBD, infectious colitis, malignancy, or celiac sprue.
- **Fecal leukocytes:** The presence of leukocytes is consistent with an inflammatory diarrhea.
- **Stool fat measurement:** The presence of excess stool fat suggests malabsorption or maldigestion as the cause of diarrhea. This can be performed by Sudan stain on a single stool specimen or a 24-hr collection while the patient consumes >100 g of fat/day. Normal fat absorption is 95% efficient, so <5 g of fat in the stool sample is normal.
- **Stool culture:** Although it is less common as a cause of chronic diarrhea, infectious diarrhea has occasionally been implicated.
- **Stool for ova and parasites:** Three samples should be sent for exam of ova and parasites.
- **Laxative screening:** This should be reserved for patients in whom the diagnosis of surreptitious laxative use is suspected.

The type of diarrhea can typically be classified based on the results of the initial evaluation and stool studies. Further diagnostic evaluation is dictated by the type of diarrhea.

Chronic Secretory Diarrhea

Patients with secretory diarrhea typically experience watery diarrhea, and stool studies reveal a normal osmotic gap. Several studies should be performed to further evaluate. Structural diseases should be excluded by endoscopic studies, including flexible sigmoidoscopy or colonoscopy and small bowel biopsy by upper endoscopy. In addition, a small bowel follow through and abdominal CT scan should be considered. Specific testing for peptide-secreting tumors should be performed if the clinical situation suggests this diagnosis. Serum levels of vasoactive intestinal peptide, gastrin, calcitonin, and urinary excretion of 5-hydroxyindoleacetic acid and histamine can be measured.

Chronic Inflammatory Diarrhea

Patients with an inflammatory disorder may have fecal leukocytes present in the stool sample. In addition, other patients may have anemia, leukocytosis, hypoalbuminemia, or occult blood in the stool. In these cases, microbiologic studies, including *C. difficile* toxin and/or colonic biopsy may be helpful, depending on the clinical scenario. Colonoscopy or flexible sigmoidoscopy may be indicated for structural evaluation or biopsy to rule out IBD.

Chronic Osmotic Diarrhea

A stool osmotic gap >125 mOsm/kg suggests osmotic diarrhea. In most patients with osmotic diarrhea, the cause is either carbohydrate malabsorption or ingestion of magnesium-containing salts. A trial of lactose-free diet should be performed, as this is the most common cause of carbohydrate malabsorption. Review all medications to evaluate for inadvertent magnesium ingestion. Finally, if surreptitious laxative use is suspected, stool analysis for laxatives and magnesium can be performed.

Chronic Steatorrhea

If stool studies suggest excess fat, then pursue evaluation for causes of malabsorption. Small bowel studies, including radiologic barium studies and endoscopic biopsies as well as tests of pancreatic insufficiency, should be performed.

Treatment

Treatment of chronic diarrhea depends on the etiology. All patients with chronic diarrhea require careful attention to volume status and electrolytes. In addition, many patients require replacement of fat-soluble vitamins, especially those with chronic steatorrhea. In some cases, chronic diarrhea is cured if the etiology is bacterial, parasitic, dietary, or related to an offending medication. An example is removing gluten-containing foods from the diets of patients with celiac sprue. The use of glucocorticoids or other antiinflammatory agents often improves diarrhea associated with IBD. In cases of ileal bile acid malabsorption, an absorptive agent such as cholestyramine is extremely helpful. The recommended dose of cholestyramine is 4 g PO tid.

When a specific etiology for chronic diarrhea is not found, empiric therapy may be helpful. In the case of mild to moderate watery diarrhea, mild opiates, such as loperamide (4 mg PO, up to 16 mg/day) or diphenoxylate plus atropine (Lomotil) (2 tabs PO qid), are often beneficial. Other, more potent options include tincture of opium and belladonna. These antimotility agents must be used with caution in IBD because of the potential complication of toxic megacolon. Finally, in cases of severe secretory diarrhea, octreotide (a somatostatin analog) may be given SC to decrease the volume of diarrhea.

KEY POINTS TO REMEMBER

- Diarrhea is generally caused by changes in water and electrolyte transport, which can occur as a result of impaired absorption, increased secretion, or both.
- Osmotic diarrhea has two clinical hallmarks that help lead to its diagnosis. First, the diarrhea ceases with fasting; second, the stool osmotic gap is abnormally elevated.
- Most cases of acute diarrhea are mild and are caused by self-limited processes, lasting <5 days. Nearly 90% of cases require no diagnostic evaluation and respond to simple rehydration therapy.

- Patients with bloody diarrhea, high fever, or systemic toxicity should not be given antidiarrheals.
- Anticholinergic agents are absolutely contraindicated in acute diarrhea due to the rare complication of toxic megacolon.
- Chronic diarrhea persists ≥ 4 wks and usually requires diagnostic evaluation. In contrast to acute diarrhea, chronic diarrhea often has a noninfectious etiology.
- Quantitative stool analysis often provides information about the severity and type of diarrhea, helping to guide further investigations.
- Secretory diarrheas typically have osmotic gaps <50 mOsm/kg, whereas osmotic diarrheas have osmotic gaps >125 mOsm/kg.
- In the case of mild to moderate watery diarrhea, mild opiates, such as loperamide or diphenoxylate, are often beneficial. Other, more potent options include tincture of opium and belladonna.

REFERENCES AND SUGGESTED READINGS

Afzalpurkar RG, Schiller LR, Little KH, et al. The self-limited nature of chronic idiopathic diarrhea. *N Engl J Med* 1992;327:1849–1852.

Bertomeu A, Ros E, Barragan V, et al. Chronic diarrhea with normal stool and colonic examinations: organic or functional? *J Clin Gastroenterol* 1991;13:531–536.

Bruckstein AH. Diagnosis and therapy of acute and chronic diarrhea. *Postgrad Med* 1989;86:151–159.

Donowitz M, Kokke FT, Saidi R. Evaluation of patients with chronic diarrhea. *N Engl J Med* 1995;332:725–729.

Eherer AJ, Fordtran JS. Fecal osmotic gap and pH in experimental diarrhea of various causes. *Gastroenterology* 1992;103:545–551.

Fine KD, Schiller LR. AGA technical review on the evaluation and management of chronic diarrhea. *Gastroenterology* 1999;116:1464–1486.

Zins BJ, Tremaine WJ, Carpenter HA. Collagenous colitis: mucosal biopsies and association with fecal leukocytes. *Mayo Clin Proc* 1995;70:430–433.

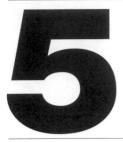

Constipation

Mukul Mehra

INTRODUCTION

There are many definitions for **constipation,** but usually the term encompasses hard, infrequent stools with difficulty in evacuation, sometimes also associated with the sense of incomplete defecation. Although the frequency of stools is variable in any given person, most epidemiologic surveys suggest that ≤ 2 stools/wk is abnormal. Studies have indicated that up to 20% of the population may have constipation at any given time. More than $400 million/yr are spent on laxatives in the United States. Management of constipation is important, as impaction may result from chronic constipation. Chronic constipation also may lead to pudendal nerve damage, fecal incontinence, or even rectal prolapse. In young women, severe constipation may cause abdominal pain leading to unnecessary appendectomy, hysterectomy, and ovarian cystectomy. Other complications, especially in the elderly, include stercoral ulcers with perforation or bleeding, volvulus, and hemorrhoids.

CAUSES

Constipation involves disordered fecal movement through the lower GI tract, namely the colon and anorectal region. Inadequate fiber and fluid intake are common precipitants. Impairment of the transit can also be due to a primary motor problem, medications, endocrine disorders, metabolic causes, structural pathology, slow transit, and pelvic floor dysfunction.

PRESENTATION

History

It is important to establish what the patient specifically means by "constipation." One must carefully elicit whether the patient has infrequent stools, hard stools, a sense of incomplete evacuation, or straining. A careful history also establishes the duration of the constipation. If present at birth, the origin is likely congenital (Hirschsprung's disease). Later onset implies acquired disorders, which can include functional constipation. It is important to elicit an adequate dietary history, including fiber and fluid intake. Associated symptoms may help narrow the differential diagnosis (Table 5-1). If the patient reports cold intolerance and weight gain, hypothyroidism must be considered. The triad of kidney stones, confusion, and constipation suggests hypercalcemia. Current diuretic use or vomiting may predispose to constipation through hypokalemia and ileus. Esophageal dysmotility along with constipation is seen in systemic sclerosis. Colon cancer may present with obstructive symptoms, and important questions include a history of weight loss, bloody stools, family history of colon cancer, and prior screening colonoscopy. Abdominal pain, bloating, and psychiatric history point toward irritable bowel syndrome. Finally, a thorough medication history must be taken, as medications are often the culprit, and discontinuation may lead to resolution of constipation without unnecessary tests.

TABLE 5-1. DIFFERENTIAL DIAGNOSIS OF CONSTIPATION

Endocrine	Diabetes mellitus, hypothyroidism, pregnancy, pheochromocytoma
Metabolic	Uremia, hypercalcemia, hypokalemia, porphyria
Neurogenic	Hirschsprung's disease, Chagas' disease, Parkinson's disease, spinal cord tumors, autonomic neuropathy, intestinal pseudoobstruction, stroke, multiple sclerosis
Collagen-vascular/smooth muscle	Scleroderma, amyloidosis, myotonic dystrophy
Structural	Colon cancer, stricture, external compression, rectocele, fissure, hemorrhoids
Medications	See Table 5-2
Other	Irritable bowel syndrome, anal spasm, rectal prolapse, depression, low-fiber diet, sedentary lifestyle, idiopathic colonic hypoactivity

Physical Exam

Auscultation for the presence and frequency of bowel sounds; palpation for presence of distention, masses, or retained stool; and exam for previous surgeries are important. The digital exam should focus on detecting sphincter tone at rest and with squeeze. Internal hemorrhoids, fissures, or masses may be found. Significant pain on rectal exam may imply a fissure. Asking the patient to strain may help the examiner discover rectal prolapse or, in a female patient, the presence of a rectocele. Gaping of the anal canal on immediate withdrawal of the finger may suggest external anal sphincter denervation. Perineal sensation should be assessed along with anal wink to assess reflex contraction of sphincter. Finally, the stool should be tested for occult blood.

MANAGEMENT

Diagnostic Evaluation

Lab tests include basic chemistry panel with glucose, calcium, and TSH. A CBC may be ordered to document anemia. More specific tests for endocrinopathies, metabolic disorders, or collagen vascular disorders should be performed only if there is a high suspicion for specific disorders. Imaging studies are often required but not always necessary. An obstructive series may indicate stool retention or megacolon or may reveal bowel obstruction. Often, a stool-filled colon is observed. Barium radiographs may be done if suspicious for megacolon/rectum or structural disease, with luminal narrowing.

Flexible sigmoidoscopy or colonoscopy is performed when there is no obvious cause for new-onset constipation, especially in patients >50 yrs. Warning symptoms or signs such as weight loss, anemia, bloody stools, family history of colon cancer, or hemoccult-positive stools should prompt a full colonoscopy to evaluate for colon cancer. Hemorrhoids may be detected as well as fissures, which may be causing pain and, thus, secondary retention of stool. Sometimes, brownish-black discoloration of the bowel mucosa is seen, termed **melanosis coli**. It is due to chronic anthraquinone laxative use (e.g., senna, cascara), suggesting long-standing constipation. A list of medications that cause constipation is found in Table 5-2.

Colonic motility tests are useful in patients with long-standing constipation if empiric treatment has been unsuccessful and the aforementioned tests have been unrevealing. In manometric studies, pressure transducers can be placed in the sigmoid colon and rectum followed by insertion and inflation of a balloon. Various pressures are recorded at different segments of the distal bowel, and the patient's symptoms are then recorded (pain, urge to expel the balloon). In irritable bowel syn-

TABLE 5-2. MEDICATIONS CAUSING CONSTIPATION

Analgesics	Narcotics, NSAIDs
Anticholinergics	Antidepressants, antihistamines, antipsychotics, antispasmodics
Cation containing	Iron, antacids (aluminum based), sucralfate, calcium-containing medicines, barium, arsenic, lead, mercury, bismuth, lithium
Other	Calcium channel blockers, pseudoephedrine

drome, patients have low compliance of the bowel wall and, thus, tolerability to the inflation of the balloon as opposed to megarectum, in which the opposite occurs. Defecography is rarely done but may identify puborectalis dysfunction, abnormal perineal descent, or rectoceles. Colonic transit studies may identify idiopathic slow-transit constipation. Radiopaque markers are ingested and transit time monitored by serial radiographs.

Treatment

Acute, short-lived constipation can usually be successfully managed with a short course of a laxative after appropriate initial evaluation to exclude obstruction. Specific management may be available if investigation reveals a treatable condition. In chronic constipation, or if a specific diagnosis is not made after investigation, several options exist for management. Dietary approaches are first-line interventions for all patients. A diet high in fiber through foods such as bran, fruits, and vegetables (beans, lentils) may be helpful. Fiber supplementation can begin at 10 g/day. It is important that the patient maintains adequate hydration. The patient should be informed about possible bloating, distention, and flatulence from increased fiber. Fiber can be increased by approximately 5 g/day each week to a total intake of approximately 25 g. Patients who cannot meet these requirements can also use methylcellulose, calcium polycarbophil, or psyllium.

Pharmacologic options may be also required. More than 700 products are available.

- **Bulk-forming laxatives** are natural or synthetic polysaccharides/cellulose derivatives that add bulk to stool by retaining water. Examples are methylcellulose, calcium polycarbophil, and psyllium. Side effects include bloating and increased gas.
- **Emollient laxatives** consist of mineral oils and docusate salts. Mineral oil penetrates the stool and softens it, whereas the docusate salts lower surface tension of stool and allow more water in the stool. Examples are docusate sodium and mineral oil. Side effects are bad taste, nausea, and lipid pneumonia if aspirated.
- **Hyperosmolar laxatives** consist of nonabsorbable sugars, such as lactulose, sorbitol, and mixed electrolyte solutions (polyethylene glycol), and work by osmotically increasing fluid in bowel lumen. Side effects are electrolyte imbalance, dehydration, and bloating.
- **Saline laxatives** create an osmotic gradient in the GI tract, bringing fluid into the bowel lumen. Examples are magnesium citrate, phosphate, or sulfate. A side effect is magnesium toxicity (avoid in renal dysfunction).
- **Stimulant laxatives** are the most frequently prescribed laxatives. They work by increasing colonic motility (anthraquinones work by increasing fluid and electrolyte content in the distal ileum and colon). Examples are senna and bisacodyl. Side effects are cathartic colon and melanosis coli (senna, cascara).
- **Enemas** using tap water, saline, mineral or cottonseed oil, and sodium phosphate cause reflex evacuation of luminal contents.

KEY POINTS TO REMEMBER

- A careful medication history should be obtained before embarking on an involved workup of constipation.

- Complications of constipation include hemorrhoids, anal fissures, rectal prolapse, ischemic colitis, volvulus, fecal impaction, stercoral ulcers, and fecal incontinence.
- Fecal impaction should be excluded before proceeding with the use of laxatives.
- The presence of warning symptoms or signs, such as weight loss, anemia, blood in stools (gross or occult), age >50 yrs, or family history of colon cancer, should prompt colonoscopy to exclude colon cancer.
- When recommending fiber intake, free water intake must be increased, or the constipation could worsen.
- Melanosis coli indicates anthraquinone laxative abuse and, likely, long-standing constipation.

REFERENCES AND SUGGESTED READINGS

Barnett JL. Approach to the patient with constipation and fecal incontinence. In: Kelley W, ed. *Textbook of internal medicine*. Philadelphia: Lippincott, 1997.

Camilleri M, Thompson WG, Fleshman JW, Pemberton JH. Clinical management of intractable constipation. *Ann Intern Med* 1994;121(7):520–528.

Prather CM, Ortiz-Camacho CP. Evaluation and treatment of constipation and fecal impaction in adults. *Mayo Clinic Proc* 1998;73(9):881–887.

Schaefer DC, Cheskin LJ. Constipation in the elderly. *Am Fam Physician* 1998;58 (4):907–914.

Wald A. Approach to the patient with constipation. In: Yamada T, ed. *Textbook of gastroenterology*. Philadelphia: Lippincott Williams & Wilkins, 1999.

Abdominal Pain

Aaron Shiels

INTRODUCTION

Abdominal pain represents one of the most common complaints for which patients seek medical attention. The ability to accurately and efficiently diagnose and treat abdominal pain is important to internists, gastroenterologists, and surgeons. Because there are hundreds of disorders that can result in the perception of pain in the abdomen, an orderly approach is critical to avoid unnecessary testing and potentially harmful delays in diagnosis.

CAUSES

Pathophysiology

There are several mechanisms by which noxious stimuli result in the sensation of pain within the abdomen. The specific characteristics for each type of pain help in identifying the underlying disease process. The two most important mechanisms of pain are parietal pain and visceral (somatic) pain. Other important mechanisms include ischemia, musculoskeletal pain, referred pain, metabolic derangements, neurogenic pain, and functional pain.

Parietal Pain

The parietal peritoneum lining the abdominal cavity is innervated by somatic nerve fibers. The pain caused by irritation of the parietal peritoneum is therefore usually well localized and lateralizes to the site of irritation. The most frequent stimulus is inflammation, often from an inflamed adjacent organ. Other stimuli that can irritate the parietal peritoneum are blood, gastric acid, or stool. The pain is constant and is worse with motion of the peritoneum. The severity of the pain depends on the specific irritating agent and the rate of development. There is often associated reflex muscle spasm of the abdominal muscles, referred to as *involuntary guarding*.

Visceral Pain

Noxious stimuli affecting the abdominal viscera result in the perception of visceral pain. It can be due to traction on the peritoneum, distention of a hollow viscus, or muscular contraction, often against an obstructed lumen. The pain fibers innervating the visceral structures are bilateral, so pain is typically perceived in the midline. As opposed to parietal pain, visceral pain is dull and poorly localized. The pain is often intermittent or colicky but may be constant. There are often associated autonomic symptoms, including nausea, vomiting, diaphoresis, or pallor.

Differential Diagnosis

The list of diagnoses that can cause abdominal pain is extensive and includes inflammatory, mechanical, ischemic, metabolic, and neurologic conditions. This emphasizes the need for a careful history and physical exam to narrow the possible diagnoses. Table 6-1 lists some of the common causes of abdominal pain.

TABLE 6-1. CAUSES OF ABDOMINAL PAIN

Inflammatory conditions	Ischemic causes
Cholecystitis	Mesenteric ischemia
Pancreatitis	Splenic infarction
Appendicitis	Testicular torsion
Diverticulitis	Ovarian cyst torsion
Hepatitis	Metabolic causes
PID	Diabetic ketoacidosis
Peptic ulcer	Uremia
Gastroenteritis	Porphyria
Spontaneous bacterial peritonitis	Lead poisoning
Acute colitis	Other causes
Pyelonephritis	Thoracic disorders
Acute cholangitis	Herpes zoster
Mechanical causes	SLE
Small or large bowel obstruction	Musculoskeletal disorders
Volvulus	Functional abdominal pain
Biliary obstruction	
Ureteral stones	
Ruptured aortic aneurysm	
Ruptured ectopic pregnancy	

PID, pelvic inflammatory disease; SLE, systemic lupus erythematosus.

PRESENTATION

A careful, detailed history and physical exam are the keys to efficient evaluation of the patient with abdominal pain. An accurate diagnosis can be made in the majority of patients with only a meticulous history and physical exam.

History

An organized approach to the history is essential. Attempts should be made to identify the onset, duration, character, location, severity, exacerbating/alleviating factors, and associated symptoms. Some general principles regarding these aspects of the history are described here.

Onset of Pain
Pain that begins abruptly suggests possible intraabdominal catastrophe, including ruptured abdominal vasculature or perforated viscus. Pain that develops rapidly over minutes suggests inflammation or obstruction of a viscus. Gradual onset over a few hours also suggests inflammation.

Duration
Pain due to irritation of the parietal peritoneum is constant, whereas obstruction of a hollow viscus results in crampy or colicky pain that waxes and wanes.

Character
Parietal pain is usually severe and well localized, whereas the pain associated with visceral noxious stimuli is dull or gnawing and poorly localized.

Location

The location of the pain is often the most important characteristic. Because the parietal peritoneum is supplied by somatic nerves, pain is perceived in the area where the peritoneum is irritated. Visceral pain is usually midline and poorly localized, but the location may provide useful information regarding the involved organ. Radiation of the pain may also help identify the affected organ. Table 6-2 lists the commonly affected organs and the corresponding perceived areas of pain.

Severity

Severe pain suggests ruptured abdominal viscus or vasculature structure. Pain that is severe in the setting of benign exam suggests mesenteric ischemia.

Exacerbating/Alleviating Factors

Pain due to inflammation of the peritoneum is worse with coughing or movement. Pain from peptic ulcer disease often improves with eating or antacids but worsens 1–2 hrs after eating.

Associated Symptoms

Nausea, vomiting, diaphoresis, hematemesis, hematochezia, melena, obstipation, hematuria, and fever may further focus the diagnostic evaluation.

Physical Exam

As with the history, an organized approach to the exam, particularly the abdominal exam, increases the likelihood of an accurate diagnosis. An exhaustive review of all the signs is beyond the scope of this chapter. However, several points deserve emphasis.

Vital Signs

Particular attention must be given to frequent hemodynamic monitoring. The presence of tachycardia or orthostatic hypotension suggests significant volume depletion and should prompt an immediate search for the underlying cause (hemorrhage, vomiting, diarrhea, third-spacing). Tachycardia may be the only sign of impending hemodynamic collapse in a patient with a vascular catastrophe. Fever suggests an inflammatory process, often infectious. Tachypnea is often the earliest sign of sepsis.

General Appearance

Much information can be determined by observation of the patient's general appearance. Patients with peritonitis often lie very still, whereas those with renal colic often writhe in bed. Patients with acute inflammatory or vascular disorders frequently appear toxic. Generalized pallor suggests severe anemia, possibly from acute blood loss.

TABLE 6-2. ORGAN INVOLVEMENT AND PERCEIVED LOCATION OF PAIN

Esophagus	Chest, epigastrium
Stomach	Epigastrium
Small intestine	Periumbilical region
Colon	Lower abdomen
Gallbladder	Right upper quadrant, radiation to scapula, shoulder, back
Liver	Right upper quadrant
Kidney or ureter	Costovertebral angle, flank, radiation to groin
Bladder	Suprapubic region
Aorta	Mid-back region

Abdominal Exam

Because many patients with acute abdominal pain are very apprehensive, it is important to take a gentle, reassuring approach to the abdominal exam. Visually inspect the abdomen for surgical scars, distention, bulging flanks, or other obvious abnormalities. Auscultate for the presence or absence of bowel sounds next. Gentle pressure with the stethoscope allows assessment of tenderness without alarming the patient. Palpate at the site furthest away from the area of pain. Peritoneal inflammation is best determined by light percussion on the abdomen, gently shaking the bed, or asking the patient to cough. "Rebound tenderness" is less specific for peritoneal inflammation. Finally, all patients with acute abdominal pain should have a rectal and pelvic (female patients) exam performed.

MANAGEMENT

Diagnostic Evaluation

As most patients with acute abdominal pain can be diagnosed with a careful history and physical exam, further diagnostic evaluation should be targeted to the clinical scenario. Excessive undirected testing increases the costs and may cause unnecessary delays in diagnosis and treatment. Specific tests deserve special mention.

Blood Tests

A CBC should be ordered in all patients to evaluate for leukocytosis or anemia. Electrolytes and liver chemistries should also be obtained. Amylase and lipase are useful for suspected pancreatic disease. Lactate levels may be helpful for suspected bowel infarction. Finally, all female patients of childbearing age should have pregnancy excluded with a urine or serum beta-hCG.

Standard Radiography

Not all patients with acute abdominal pain require plain or upright films of the abdomen. However, abdominal x-rays are useful for diagnosing perforated viscus (identified as free air under the diaphragm), ileus, or bowel obstruction. Abdominal films are relatively safe and inexpensive and can usually be performed quickly.

Ultrasonography

Transabdominal U/S is useful for patients with suspected biliary tract disease, including acute cholecystitis, biliary pain, and choledocholithiasis. It also allows rapid diagnosis of abdominal aortic aneurysms. Its sensitivity and specificity, however, are limited by operator and interpreter experience. U/S is safe and can be performed at the bedside in most cases.

Computed Tomography

Abdominal CT, especially with rapid spiral scanning techniques, provides a powerful imaging tool. It allows "three-dimensional" imaging of the entire abdomen and pelvis and is less operator dependent than U/S. It is the most sensitive test for identifying perforated viscus and is useful for suspected cases of bowel obstruction, intraabdominal abscess, appendicitis, ruptured aortic aneurysm, necrotizing pancreatitis, and diverticulitis. However, care must be used in selecting patients for abdominal CT. The test is time-consuming and costly and may unnecessarily delay diagnosis and treatment, especially in patients who require urgent surgery. In addition, it carries risk of anaphylactic reaction or nephrotoxicity from contrast dye.

KEY POINTS TO REMEMBER

- A careful, detailed history and physical exam are the keys to efficient evaluation of the patient with abdominal pain. An accurate diagnosis can be made in the majority of patients with only a meticulous history and physical exam.
- The pain caused by irritation of the parietal peritoneum is usually well localized and lateralizes to the site of irritation.

- Visceral pain is dull and poorly localized. There are often associated autonomic symptoms, including nausea, vomiting, diaphoresis, or pallor.
- Peritoneal inflammation is best determined by light percussion on the abdomen, gently shaking the bed, or asking the patient to cough. "Rebound tenderness" is less specific for peritoneal inflammation.

REFERENCES AND SUGGESTED READINGS

Fauci A, ed. *Harrison's principles of internal medicine*, 14th ed. New York: McGraw-Hill, 1998:65–68.

Sleisenger MH, Fordtran JS. *Gastrointestinal disease: pathophysiology, diagnosis, management,* 5th ed. Philadelphia: WB Saunders, 1993:150–162.

Wolfe MM. *Therapy of digestive disorders.* Philadelphia: WB Saunders, 2000:711–716.

Upper Gastrointestinal Bleeding

Rajesh Shah

INTRODUCTION

Upper GI (UGI) bleeding is generally defined as bleeding that occurs in the digestive tract proximal to the ligament of Treitz. It is a significant cause of morbidity and mortality in the United States. Recent studies have estimated the yearly hospitalization rate due to UGI bleeding at approximately 100/100,000 persons with nearly half of these hospitalizations occurring in patients >60 yrs. Mortality rates range from 3.5% to 7%, accounting for between 10,000 and 20,000 deaths in the United States annually. It should be noted that approximately 80% of all acute episodes of UGI hemorrhage resolve without intervention and require supportive care only. Thus, the consultant must place emphasis on determining which patients require intervention to stop bleeding or prevent rebleeding. This emphasis has led to the development of scoring systems that attempt to predict risk and outcomes. A number of factors, including age, comorbidity, presence of shock, etiology, and presence of major stigmata of bleeding, have been used. The advent of esophagogastroduodenal endoscopy has allowed clinicians to diagnose with certainty the etiology of hemorrhage, predict accurately the risk of rebleeding, and provide therapeutic intervention when indicated. It is estimated that >90% of patients admitted for UGI bleeding undergo upper endoscopy within 24 hrs. These advancements, which are discussed in greater detail below, have led to a significant reduction both in the length and cost of hospital stay.

CAUSES

Pathophysiology

Nearly 80% of all UGI bleeding episodes (including variceal hemorrhage) require only supportive care. Pathophysiology of UGI bleeding depends greatly on the etiology of the bleed, but characteristic clinical manifestations are produced when blood enters the digestive tract.

Hematemesis, the vomiting of blood, is commonly the cardinal manifestation of UGI hemorrhage. It invariably indicates bleeding above the ligament of Treitz. When vomitus is red, recent bleeding should be suspected. However, when blood is present in the digestive tract for a longer period of time, it becomes subject to acid degradation within the stomach and the classic "coffee ground emesis" is produced.

Melena describes black, tarry, sticky stool with a characteristic odor and is produced when blood is digested. It signifies bleeding in the digestive tract anywhere from the esophagus to the ascending colon but is most commonly seen in UGI bleeding. As little as 60 cc of blood can result in a single melenic stool. It should be noted that only half of patients with melena have concurrent hematemesis, whereas almost all patients with hematemesis have subsequent melena.

Hematochezia, or bright red blood per rectum, usually denotes bleeding distal to the ligament of Treitz. However, brisk UGI bleeding can produce hematochezia. In a recent series, 11% of patients with hematochezia were later found to have a lesion in the UGI tract. Patients with UGI bleeding resulting in hematochezia are invariably hemodynamically unstable, often with profound hypovolemic shock.

Persistent UGI hemorrhage may eventually lead to depletion of intravascular volume. *Orthostatic hypotension*, defined as a 10-mm decrease in systolic BP when going from supine to upright position, denotes a 20% loss of intravascular volume. Severe, rapid, or unrelenting bleeding may produce shock (approximately 40% loss of volume) with the resultant signs of tachycardia, supine hypotension, and pallor. However, increased vagal tone to the heart caused by shock may produce bradycardia and confuse the clinical picture. Concomitant use of beta-adrenergic antagonists may also mask the tachycardia that would normally be seen with intravascular depletion.

Ischemic organ damage can be precipitated by ongoing blood loss. The clinician must in particular be mindful of cardiac ischemia induced by severe anemia. Pulmonary aspiration is an occasional complication of hematemesis. Patients with advanced liver disease and variceal bleeding are particularly prone to aspiration.

Differential Diagnosis

Common Causes

PEPTIC ULCER DISEASE. Peptic ulcer disease is the most common cause of UGI hemorrhage. Risk factors include *Helicobacter pylori* infection, NSAIDs, physiologic stress, and hypersecretion of gastric acid, as in Zollinger-Ellison syndrome. Bleeding may occur without previous symptoms of dyspepsia and usually occurs when the ulcer erodes into the wall of a vessel. Ulcers located on the lesser curve of the stomach and the posteroinferior wall of the duodenal bulb have been demonstrated to rebleed with greater frequency.

GASTRIC EROSIONS. Gastric erosions are most commonly related to NSAID or ASA use. An *erosion* can be defined as a 3- to 5-mm break in the mucosa that does not cross the muscularis mucosa. Erosions should be distinguished from gastritis (either chronic or acute), which is a histologic diagnosis and does not cause significant hemorrhage. ASA and NSAIDs have been shown to cause hemorrhagic gastropathy in normal subjects within 24 hrs of administration. This bleeding is generally not severe and is always self-limiting. Portal gastropathy caused by alcoholic cirrhosis may be a mechanism of nonvariceal bleeding in alcoholics. Erythema, petechiae, multiple bleeding areas, vascular ectasias, and congestion are the hallmarks of portal gastropathy.

VARICEAL HEMORRHAGE. Variceal hemorrhage most commonly occurs with esophageal varices but can also be seen with gastric and duodenal varices. Varices may be seen in patients who have portal HTN of any cause. However, the vast majority of patients have underlying liver cirrhosis. In the United States, alcoholic cirrhosis is the most common cause of portal HTN. Approximately one-third of patients with cirrhosis have at least one variceal hemorrhage. Up to 50% of patients who have cirrhosis and present with UGI bleed have a source of bleeding other than varices. The portosystemic gradient must be >12 mm Hg for varices to form, but higher pressures do not appear to increase the risk of rupture. Red or blue color and larger size of the varix predict a greater risk of rupture and subsequent hemorrhage. Mortality from a single variceal bleed is approximately 30%. 60–70% of patients who survive the initial episode die within 1 yr. This high mortality rate is due not only to the high risk of rebleeding (60–70%), but also to the comorbid conditions that patients with varices often have. Gastric varices may occur in the setting of portal HTN or after injection sclerotherapy of esophageal varices. Isolated gastric varices may be seen with splenic vein thrombosis. Bleeding risk is similar to that of esophageal varices.

MALLORY-WEISS TEAR. Tears generally are preceded by prolonged episodes of retching or vomiting (typically after an alcohol binge). They occur most often at the gastroesophageal junction and are evidenced by longitudinal ulcerations. Bleeding ensues when an underlying venous or arterial plexus is exposed by the tear. Hemorrhage may be brisk but is self-limited, and the tear usually heals within a few days. Continued vomiting, however, can lead to esophageal rupture (Boerhaave's syndrome). Comorbid portal HTN confers a risk of more massive bleeding from Mallory-Weiss tears.

Uncommon Causes

- Esophagitis can be due to reflux disease, infection (*Candida*, herpes simplex, CMV), radiation therapy, or medications (quinidine, tetracycline, alendronate) but rarely causes severe bleeding.
- Arteriovenous malformations include Dieulafoy's lesion (an ectatic vessel that erodes through the mucosa), hemorrhagic telangiectasias (seen in Osler-Weber-Rendu syndrome), and those associated with chronic renal failure.
- *Gastric antral vascular ectasia* is also known as "watermelon stomach." This condition results in a classic linear erythematous gastric pattern.
- Aortoenteric fistulas generally occur after aortic surgery involving Dacron grafts and usually involve the third part of the duodenum. However, they may occur anywhere in the GI tract and are often very difficult to identify. The classic "herald bleed" can occur days to weeks before massive fatal hemorrhage.
- Hemobilia is hemorrhage into the biliary tract, usually caused by trauma.
- Hemosuccus pancreaticus is hemorrhage into the pancreatic duct and usually occurs in patients with chronic pancreatitis, pseudocysts, or trauma.

PRESENTATION

History

A careful history should include history of hematemesis, melena, or hematochezia. Use of color-coded cards is helpful in determining the actual color of the stools. Abdominal pain can help localize the source of bleeding or direct the clinician toward other diagnoses. A history of chronic abdominal pain or dyspeptic symptoms points toward peptic ulcer disease. Liver disease and chronic alcohol use are important risk factors for variceal hemorrhage. A history of vomiting and retching suggests a Mallory-Weiss tear. Other important points in the medical history include surgeries (especially aortic graft surgery), trauma, coagulation disorders, malignancies, and immune status. A careful medication history should be taken, with particular emphasis on NSAIDs, ASA, and oral anticoagulants.

Physical Exam

Vital signs are the most important aspect of the physical exam. Tachycardia and hypotension suggest a hemodynamically significant bleed that requires prompt diagnosis and therapy. Stigmata of chronic liver disease and portal HTN (i.e., telangiectasias, ascites, splenomegaly) should be closely evaluated. Abdominal tenderness may be present in peptic ulcer disease. Digital rectal exam can provide useful information as to color and consistency of stools, thus directing the clinician toward a UGI or lower GI source.

MANAGEMENT

Resuscitation

Evaluation for possible causes of hemorrhage is performed during or after hemodynamic stabilization. Signs of hypovolemia (i.e., hypotension, tachycardia, pallor, agitation) necessitate immediate repletion of intravascular volume.

Intravascular volume should be restored initially with either isotonic saline or lactated Ringer's solution. Two large-bore ($\geq$ 18-gauge) IV lines should be in place at all times. Centrally inserted triple lumen catheters do not confer any advantage over peripheral IVs in terms of rate of fluid administration. Vasopressors should be avoided, as hypotension is secondary to hypovolemia. Rate of IV fluid administration is dictated by the degree of hypovolemia. Rarely, patients bleed at a rate such that special equipment (so-called rapid-infuser) may be required to keep up with blood loss.

Blood transfusion with packed red cells is the method of choice for volume resuscitation in patients with severe UGI hemorrhage. All patients who are admitted for GI bleeding should be typed and crossed, and crossmatched blood should be transfused when possible. However, in the case of catastrophic bleeding, O-negative units should be used without delay. The target Hct is 25%, although in patients with coronary disease, a Hct of 30% is desirable. Care must be taken not to overtransfuse patients with variceal hemorrhage due to the risk of inducing hemorrhage from overdistending the varices. Coagulopathy should be corrected with FFP in the unstable patient, but vitamin K (5–10 mg SC) can be used if the patient is hemodynamically stable. Heparin drips should be discontinued and protamine used for reversal if necessary. If the patient is at risk for aspiration, endotracheal intubation to protect the airway should be considered. It is often required for management of variceal bleeding.

Lab Evaluation

A CBC is the most important initial lab test. Hemoglobin and Hct must be followed through the entire hospital stay. Initial Hct does not reflect the amount of blood loss because blood volume is contracted. Once blood volume is restored, usually in the form of IV fluid administration, Hct begins to fall. Platelet transfusions are given if the platelet count is <50,000 cells/μL. Basic metabolic panels may demonstrate a BUN elevated out of proportion to creatinine. This is due both to hypovolemia and to increased absorption of blood. PT and aPTT should be checked initially, and coagulopathy should be corrected.

Nasogastric Lavage

Positive gastric aspirate indicates that bleeding has occurred proximal to the jejunum. Negative aspirate does not preclude UGI bleeding. An aspirate is considered positive if fresh blood or "coffee ground" material is present. There is no utility in testing for occult blood (gastroccult) in gastric aspirate. NG lavage serves two purposes. First, it can be used to assess rapidity and severity of bleeding by determining how much water is required to clear the aspirate. Second, it clears the endoscopic field of blood, clots, and particulate matter, thus ensuring clear visualization and facilitating accurate diagnosis and treatment. The NG tube does not need to be left in place, especially if bleeding is not brisk and the lavage rapidly clears with water or saline.

Upper Endoscopy

Esophagogastroduodenoscopy is the preferred method for evaluating patients with UGI bleeding. Endoscopy allows direct visualization of the mucosa and identification of the bleeding site. Early endoscopy (i.e., within 24 hrs of admission) has not been demonstrated to decrease mortality. However, total cost, length of hospitalization, and need for emergent surgery have all been greatly reduced, largely due to the therapeutic options available to the endoscopist. It is important that the hemodynamically unstable patient be adequately volume resuscitated and any coagulopathy be corrected before performing upper endoscopy. Morbidity and mortality from upper endoscopy have been reported at 1% and 0.1%, respectively. Contraindications include an agitated patient, perforated viscus, and severe cardiopulmonary disease. Definitive diagnosis is made when active bleeding, stigmata of bleeding, or significant lesions are seen. 24% of patients with melena have no diagnosis by upper endoscopy.

Other Studies

Arteriography is rarely indicated but can be helpful in localizing the source of bleeding if blood loss into the GI tract is too brisk to allow for endoscopy. The rate of the bleed must be >0.5 cc/min. Selective abdominal arteriography in the hands of a skilled radiologist also allows for therapeutic capabilities in the form of arterial embolization. In some situations, the bleeding is so brisk that emergent surgery or transjugular intrahepatic portosystemic shunt (TIPS; in the case of variceal bleeding) is the only option for management.

Treatment

Peptic Ulcer Disease

Appropriate therapy is dictated by findings at endoscopy. Table 7-1 gives the rebleeding rates after medical therapy of various endoscopic stigmata of hemorrhage. IV H_2-antagonists have not been shown to reduce surgery or mortality rates in patients with UGI hemorrhage. A recent study demonstrated significant reduction in surgery and mortality when patients at high risk for rebleeding were given high-dose proton pump inhibitors (PPIs) (omeprazole, 40 mg PO bid for 5 days). The study did not include patients with visible arterial spurting, nor was endoscopic therapy performed.

Ulcers that demonstrate arterial spurting or a visible vessel generally should be treated endoscopically. Thermal coagulation and injection therapy with epinephrine have both been shown to achieve hemostasis and decrease rebleeding rates. Combination therapy appears to further reduce rebleeding. Some endoscopists attempt to dislodge adherent clots, so that an underlying vessel can be treated endoscopically. Patients with low-risk ulcers (i.e., clean base) may be discharged and followed on an outpatient basis. IV PPIs have recently been shown to decrease rebleeding rates in patients who have already undergone endoscopic therapy. However, IV PPIs may be unnecessary and expensive in patients who can tolerate oral PPIs.

Surgery is reserved for patients with intractable hemorrhage, recurrent bleeding despite repeated attempts at endoscopic therapy, or blood types that are difficult to crossmatch. Arterial embolization by selective arterial catheterization is an alternative for patients too unstable to undergo surgery.

Variceal Hemorrhage

Octreotide acetate is a long-acting somatostatin analog that reduces portal pressure, thus improving hemostasis when used in conjunction with endoscopic therapy. It should be started immediately in any patient with suspected variceal hemorrhage. It is given as a 50- to 100-μg IV bolus followed by an infusion at 25–50 μg/hr. Vasopressin was formerly used as medical treatment of variceal hemorrhage but has been replaced by octreotide due to its cardiovascular side effects.

Sclerotherapy involves injection of a variety of sclerosing agents (ethanolamine oleate, sodium tetradecyl sulfate, polidocanol, morrhuate sodium, or ethanol) directly into the varix and achieves hemostasis in >90% of cases. However, recurrent bleeding within 10 days occurs in up to 50% of patients, and side effects of therapy include fever, ulceration, strictures, perforation, ARDS, and sepsis. Endoscopic variceal ligation, which involves banding of the base of the varix, has largely replaced injection sclerotherapy in acute variceal hemorrhage. Endoscopic variceal ligation is easier to perform endoscopically and has been shown to reduce rebleeding, complications, and mortality.

Balloon tamponade should only be employed when hemorrhage is uncontrollable or when urgent endoscopy is not available. The Sengstaken-Blakemore tube and the

TABLE 7-1. ULCER REBLEEDING RISK BASED ON ENDOSCOPIC APPEARANCE

Endoscopic finding	Risk of rebleeding (%)
Arterial spurting	90
Visible vessel	50
Adherent clot	25
Oozing without visible vessel	10–20
Pigment spot	7–10
Clean-based ulcer	3–5

Minnesota tube, both of which have gastric and esophageal balloons, are commonly used. Hemostasis is achieved 70–90% of the time. Complications can be severe and include esophageal perforation, aspiration, chest pain, erosion, agitation, and death due to asphyxiation.

TIPS is reserved for patients with intractable variceal bleeding. It creates a direct portosystemic shunt, thereby decreasing pressure within the portal vein. Technical success is achieved >90% of the time, but complications include hepatic encephalopathy in up to 25% of patients, shunt stenosis, and rebleeding. Surgical shunts are rarely used due to the availability of TIPS procedures. Portacaval and distal splenorenal shunts achieve hemostasis 95% of the time but are associated with mortality rates of 50–80%, largely due to severe underlying liver disease.

Mallory-Weiss Tear
Endoscopic treatment is only employed when tears involve active and ongoing bleeding. Epinephrine injection and thermal coagulation are both efficacious in controlling hemorrhage. Sclerosants should be avoided due to risk of further tearing or perforation. PPIs can promote healing after the acute episode.

Gastric Erosions
Management is directed at primary prevention. In the ICU, IV H_2-receptor blockers or oral PPIs are used to prevent stress ulceration. PPIs have replaced misoprostol for use in patients who require continued NSAID therapy.

KEY POINTS TO REMEMBER

- Peptic ulcer disease accounts for nearly half of all UGI bleeding episodes.
- UGI bleeding is self-limited in almost 80% of cases.
- A negative NG aspirate does not preclude UGI bleeding.
- Ulcers with a clean base are at low risk for rebleeding; therefore, patients may be safely discharged with outpatient follow-up.
- Ulcers with active arterial spurting or a visible vessel are at high risk for rebleeding and should be treated endoscopically.
- Mortality from a single episode of variceal bleeding is 30%, with 60–70% of patients dying within 1 yr.
- The portosystemic gradient must exceed 12 mm Hg for varices to form, but there is no correlation between portal pressure and risk of rupture.
- Whereas one-third of patients with cirrhosis have at least one variceal bleed, up to 50% of cirrhotics who present with UGI bleeding have a source other than varices.
- Variceal band ligation has replaced sclerotherapy in acute variceal hemorrhage.

REFERENCES AND SUGGESTED READINGS

Cook D, Guyatt G, Salena B, et al. Endoscopic therapy for acute nonvariceal upper gastrointestinal hemorrhage: a meta-analysis. *Gastroenterology* 1992;102:139–148.

Freeman M, Cass O, Peine C, et al. The non-bleeding visible vessel versus the sentinel clot: natural history and risk of rebleeding. *Gastrointest Endosc* 1993;39:359–366.

Morrissey JF, Reichelderfer M. Gastrointestinal endoscopy. *N Engl J Med* 1991;325:1142–1149 and 1214–1222.

Rockey DC, Auslander A, Greenberg PD. Detection of upper gastrointestinal blood with fecal occult blood tests. *Am J Gastroenterol* 1999;94:344–350.

Rollhauser C, Fleischer D. Nonvariceal upper gastrointestinal bleeding: an update. *Endoscopy* 1997;29:91–105.

Silverstein F, Gilbert D, Tedesco F, et al. The national ASGE survey on upper gastrointestinal bleeding. *Gastrointest Endosc* 1981;27:73–79.

Zuccaro G. Bleeding peptic ulcer: pathogenesis and endoscopic therapy. *Gastroenterol Clin North Am* 1993;22:737–750.

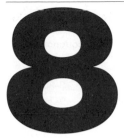

Lower Gastrointestinal Bleeding

Sandeep K. Tripathy

INTRODUCTION

Definition

Lower GI bleeding is defined as bleeding originating distal to the ligament of Treitz. Lower GI bleeds have also been referred to as **bright red blood per rectum, maroon stools,** and **hematochezia.** The severity of lower GI bleeding runs the spectrum from patients with scant but frequent passages of blood per rectum with no major changes in their hemoglobin to massive hemorrhage for which urgent decisions for surgery or other life-saving interventions must be made.

Patients with lower GI bleeding are less likely to present with shock or orthostasis as compared to patients with upper GI bleeding. They also tend to present with higher initial hemoglobin and are less likely to require a blood transfusion as compared to patients with upper GI bleeds.

Epidemiology

Unlike upper GI bleeding, lower GI bleeding tends to be slow and intermittent. Several studies have revealed that the incidence of lower GI bleeds is much less than that of upper GI bleeds (anywhere from one-fifth to one-third as frequent). The annual incidence rate of lower GI bleed is 20–27 cases/100,000 (in contrast to upper GI bleed, in which the annual incidence is reported to be 100–200 cases/100,000). It is important to realize, however, that the majority of patients with an acute GI bleed (upper or lower tract) pass blood, in some form, from their rectum. Lower GI bleeds have been found more significantly in men than in women. They are also more common with increasing age (there is a >200-fold increase from the third to ninth decades). This is primarily due to the age-related increase of diverticulosis and angiodysplasia (the two major causes of acute lower GI bleeds). Overall mortality rates from lower GI bleeds is <5%. Historically, this is lower than mortality rates of patients with upper GI bleeds. It should be noted that in most series, lower GI bleeding was rarely the cause of death. As is the case with upper GI bleeding, 80% of bleeding episodes resolve spontaneously. Among the patients in whom bleeding ceases, 25% have recurrent bleeding.

CAUSES

Differential Diagnosis

The two major causes of acute lower GI bleeding are diverticular bleeding and angiodysplasia (Table 8-1). The most common causes of chronic lower GI bleeding are hemorrhoids and colonic neoplasia.

Diverticular Bleeding

Diverticular bleeding is the most common cause of major lower GI hemorrhage due to the high prevalence of diverticulosis in the Western world. Bleeding occurs in only 3% of patients with diverticulosis. Diverticula are usually located in the colonic wall at the sites of penetration of nutrient vessels. Bleeding presumably results from rupture of a colonic artery into the diverticular sac. Diverticular bleeding presents with acute,

TABLE 8-1.   LESIONS ENCOUNTERED IN EVALUATION OF LOWER GI BLEEDING

Lesion	Frequency (%)
Diverticular disease	17–40
Colonic vascular ectasia	2–30
Colitis (ischemic, infectious, inflammatory bowel disease, radiation)	9–21
Colonic neoplasm/postpolypectomy	4–10
Anorectal source	4–10
Upper GI source	0–11
Small bowel site	2–9

painless, maroon to bright red hematochezia, although melenic stools may occur. Among the 75–80% of patients in whom bleeding ceases, 25–35% have repeated episodes of diverticular hemorrhage. If the initial bleeding ceases spontaneously, no further therapy is indicated because bleeding does not recur in most patients.

Angiodysplasias
Angiodysplasias are common causes of acute major lower GI hemorrhage and slow, intermittent blood loss. Angiodysplastic lesions are usually multiple, <5 mm in diameter, and involve primarily the cecum and right colon. Most vascular ectasias are degenerative lesions associated with aging. Two-thirds of patients with colonic angiodysplasia are >70 yrs. The pathogenesis of angiodysplasias is unknown, but one theory is that repeated, partial, intermittent obstruction of the submucosal veins where they pierce the muscle layers of the colon leads to dilation and tortuosity of the veins. Eventually, the entire arteriolar-capillar-venular unit dilates, creating a small arteriovenous communication. Because active bleeding is infrequently identified, and because these lesions appear to be common in the elderly without a significant blood loss history, definitive diagnosis is difficult. If no other source of GI bleeding is identified in a patient with recurrent or persistent GI bleeding sufficient to require transfusions or cause significant anemia, the presence of angiodysplasia is an indication for treatment. The diagnosis of vascular ectasias can be made by colonoscopy or angiography. Both diagnostic modalities frequently identify the lesions without demonstrating active bleeding. The diagnostic sensitivity of colonoscopy is 80%, with a 90% specificity. The earliest angiographic sign is a densely opacified, dilated, tortuous, slowly emptying intramural vein. A vascular tuft represents a more advanced lesion, and an early-filling vein reflects an arteriovenous communication and is a late sign.

Benign and Malignant Neoplasms
Benign and malignant neoplasms of the colon are common lesions that occur predominantly in the elderly. Major hemorrhage from a colonic polyp or carcinoma is uncommon. The diagnosis is made by colonoscopy or barium enema, and treatment is colonoscopic or surgical excision, as appropriate.

Hemorrhoids and Anal Fissures
Hemorrhoids and anal fissures are probably the most common causes of minor intermittent lower GI bleeding. The characteristic clinical history of hemorrhoidal bleeding is bright red blood on the toilet tissue or around the stool but not mixed in the stool. Bleeding often occurs with straining or passage of hard stool. A similar history is common in patients with bleeding from anal fissures, with the exception that anal fissures are often painful. Only rarely is the amount of bleeding severe enough to cause iron-deficient anemia or acute and severe enough to require transfusions. Massive hemorrhage from simple hemorrhoids is rare but may occur from rectal varices in patients with portal HTN. Perianal disease is treated with sitz baths, bulk-forming

agents, avoidance of straining, and ointments or suppositories. It is unknown if actual therapeutic benefit is obtained with locally applied medications containing lubricants and hydrocortisone, but many patients report symptomatic relief. When bleeding or other symptoms continue to be troublesome, hemorrhoidal banding, coagulation techniques, or surgery may be indicated.

Meckel's Diverticulum
Meckel's diverticulum is the most frequent congenital anomaly of the intestinal tract, with an incidence of 0.3–3.0% in autopsy reports. It develops from incomplete obliteration of the vitelline duct, leaving an ileal diverticulum. Patients present with painless bleeding that may be melenic or bright red, although its appearance is classically described as "currant jelly." The diagnosis can be made by radiolabeled technetium scanning. Barium filling of the diverticulum may occur, especially with an enteroclysis. Mesenteric angiography may demonstrate the site of bleeding. Surgical excision is the treatment of choice.

Inflammatory Bowel Disease
Inflammatory bowel disease usually causes a small to moderate degree of bleeding, although it rarely may be massive. The blood is usually mixed in with the stool and is associated with other symptoms of the disease, such as diarrhea, tenesmus, and pain. The diagnosis and treatment of this bleeding depend on the management of the underlying disorder.

Ischemic Colitis
Ischemic colitis is a common entity in the elderly population. It is usually caused by "low-flow states" and small vessel disease rather than large vessel occlusion. Any segment of the colon may be involved, although the most common are the splenic flexure, descending colon, and sigmoid colon. The typical presentation is mild, crampy abdominal pain localized to the lower left side, followed within 24 hrs by rectal bleeding or bloody diarrhea. The blood loss is characteristically minimal, although massive bleeding has rarely been described. Plain abdominal films may show the classic "thumbprinting" lesion of the colon. The diagnosis is best made by colonoscopy and biopsy. Most cases resolve spontaneously with observation and medical support. Surgery is reserved for the rare circumstance of clinical deterioration with fever and rising leukocyte count or persistent hemorrhage.

Infectious Colitis
Infectious colitis caused by *Campylobacter jejuni*, *Shigella* species, invasive *Escherichia coli* or *E. coli* O157:H7, or *Clostridium difficile* often presents with bloody diarrhea. The degree of blood loss is rarely significant. The diagnosis is made by sigmoidoscopy with biopsy and stool culture. Treatment is determined by the specific pathogen.

Radiation Colopathy
Radiation colopathy is a chronic or recurrent problem that may follow irradiation immediately or present several years later. The blood loss is rarely massive but may cause iron deficiency or intermittent blood transfusions. The diagnosis is made by the history of irradiation and with endoscopic biopsy confirmation.

Colonic Ulcers
Colonic ulcers are increasingly recognized as causes of acute lower GI bleeding. Although not classically associated with colonic ulcer, NSAIDs can cause discrete ulcers throughout the colon.

Intussusception
Intussusception may present with maroon stools and is almost always accompanied by crampy abdominal pain. Uncommon in adults, it usually has a leading point, such as a polyp or malignancy. The diagnosis may be suggested by plain abdominal films and a sausage-shaped mass found during physical exam. Barium enema may be useful for

diagnosis; in children, it may be used for therapeutic reduction. Treatment of intussusception in adults is usually surgical.

Aortoenteric Fistulas

Aortoenteric fistulas are most commonly located in the third part of the duodenum but may occur anywhere in the GI tract, especially in patients who have had prior vascular surgery. Secondary fistulas have been described to the distal small bowel and colon.

PRESENTATION

History

- Clues to severity of bleeding include duration of bleeding, stool color, stool frequency, and stool volume. Abrupt hematochezia (within 24 hrs of presentation) associated with hemodynamic instability or bleeding that has occurred over several days that causes the patient to complain of dizziness or other orthostatic symptoms suggests major blood loss and the need for quick resuscitation.
- Associated symptoms, including abdominal pain, recent change in bowel habits, fever, or weight loss, may point to specific diagnoses. A recent history of anorexia or weight loss may indicate an underlying malignancy.
- Relevant medical history includes previous bleeding (diverticulosis, hemorrhoids, ulcers, varices, and angiodysplasia), recent polypectomy, past abdominal surgeries, inflammatory bowel disease, and history of radiation therapy to the abdomen or pelvis.
- Current medications should be reviewed, with particular attention to NSAIDs, ASA, and anticoagulants.
- The presence or absence of chest pain, palpitations, dyspnea on exertion, lightheadedness, or orthostatic symptoms should be determined.

Physical Exam

The physical exam should include vital signs, evaluation for orthostatic hypotension (increase in pulse by 10 bpm or decrease in systolic BP by 10 mm Hg with postural change), cardiopulmonary exam, abdominal exam, and digital rectal exam. The digital rectal exam is to inspect stool and assess for hemorrhoids or masses. Use of a standardized color chart can avoid confusion when describing the color of the stool.

MANAGEMENT

Lab Evaluation

Initial studies should include a CBC, serum electrolytes, coagulation profile, and type and crossmatch. Remember that the initial hemoglobin value may not reflect the degree of blood loss due to volume contraction. Patients >50 yrs, patients who have a history of heart disease, or patients who report chest pain/palpitations with the bleeding episode should have an ECG.

Diagnostic Procedures

- **NG lavage** should be performed if the possibility of an upper GI source exists. Almost without exception, patients with upper GI bleeding and hematochezia are hemodynamically unstable, often with hypovolemic shock. If suspicion of upper GI bleeding remains despite a negative NG lavage, then upper endoscopy should be performed.
- **Colonoscopy** is the most frequently used diagnostic tool for evaluating lower GI bleeding. Successful colonoscopy requires timing the procedure to completion of adequate bowel preparation. Rapid lavage preparation (instillation of 2–3 L poly-

ethylene glycol solution via NG tube over 1–2 hrs) followed by colonoscopy after the solution has been placed leaves the colon very clean, allowing for identification of active bleeding. It is important that the patient is adequately volume resuscitated and hemodynamically stable before the bowel preparation is initiated. The overall diagnostic yield of colonoscopy is 70–80%. Because of increased risk of perforation as the endoscope passes through poorly visualized areas, extreme care must be taken in patients with massive bleeding or suboptimal preparation. In these cases, other procedures may be used as an alternative.

- **Tagged RBC scan** may be used in the evaluation of active lower GI bleed. Bleeding must exceed a rate of 0.1 mL/min. The procedure is of very low risk. However, the test is positive < half of the time. One use of this procedure is as a screening test before angiography. A patient with a negative tagged RBC scan is unlikely to have a positive angiogram.
- **Angiography** offers accurate diagnosis and therapy in the rapidly bleeding patient. Bleeding rates of 0.5–1 mL/min are required to detect extravasation into the bowel from a bleeding site. The overall diagnostic yield from arteriography ranges from 40–78%. If a bleeding source is identified, therapeutic modalities can be used to stop bleeding (including injection of vasopressin or selective embolization). Complications of this procedure include contrast allergy, bleeding from arterial puncture, and embolism from dislodged thrombus. Arteriography should be reserved for those patients with massive, ongoing bleeding for which colonoscopy is not feasible.

Treatment

Resuscitation of the patient is the initial step in patient management. (See Chap. 7, Resuscitation, p. 33 for details on acute resuscitation.) Most patients in whom bleeding ceases require elective treatment of the source of bleeding depending on diagnosis. Urgent therapeutic maneuvers are indicated for patients requiring transfusion of more than 3 U of red cells.

Therapeutic Colonoscopy

Endoscopic therapy involves the uses of thermal coagulation (heater probe, bipolar/multipolar coagulation, laser therapy), injection of vasoconstrictors, and injection of sclerosants. Placement of metallic hemoclips has also been successful in the treatment of diverticular bleeding. Approximately 25% of patients with lower GI bleeds have lesions that are amenable to endoscopic therapy (angiodysplasia, diverticular bleeding with visible vessels, bleeding polypectomy sites, some colonic ulcers).

Intraarterial Vasopressin

Intraarterial vasopressin is effective in controlling hemorrhage from diverticula and angiodysplasia. In patients with persistent bleeding, vasopressin should be infused after selective catheterization of the bleeding vessels. Repeat contrast injection at 15–30 mins should confirm cessation of the hemorrhage. The complication rate of vasopressin infusion is 5–15% and includes cardiovascular toxicity and problems associated with an indwelling catheter. Patients who do not respond to vasopressin therapy may require surgery or embolization. Patients receiving embolotherapy are at risk of developing the serious complication of bowel infarction. Lesser degrees of ischemia are more common. For these reasons, embolization techniques should be used as a last resort in patients who are poor surgical candidates. Older patients who develop lower GI bleeding may be at greater risk for ischemic complications from embolic therapy because of diffuse arteriosclerosis.

Surgical Therapy

As with upper GI bleeding, surgery should not be postponed excessively in the patient with persistent lower GI bleeding because morbidity and mortality increase with delay. Prior surgical practice included left hemicolectomy for lower GI bleeding and was associated with high rebleeding rates. Better preop localization improves postop rebleeding rates. The surgical mortality rates for recent series are 5–10%.

For the difficult situation of recurrent massive bleeding without demonstration of a bleeding site, a subtotal colectomy may be indicated in patients with good overall prognoses.

KEY POINTS TO REMEMBER

* Initiate resuscitative measures and appropriate level of monitoring before starting diagnostic testing and therapeutic intervention. Intensive care monitoring is appropriate for patients with unstable vital signs (not responding to resuscitative therapy) and those with comorbid conditions.
* Upper GI bleeding source must be considered. An NG aspirate that reveals bile and is negative for blood makes an upper GI source less likely. Upper endoscopy should be performed if there is evidence of blood in the NG aspirate or if NG aspirate is negative and an upper source is suspected.
* Endoscopy (colonoscopy or sigmoidoscopy) is the test of choice for structural evaluation of lower GI bleed.
* Arteriography should be reserved for patients with massive, ongoing bleeding that makes endoscopy unfeasible or when colonoscopy does not reveal a source of bleeding.
* Patients with persistent or recurrent lower GI bleeding may require surgical intervention. The accurate localization of bleeding before surgery decreases morbidity and mortality.
* In cases of lower GI bleeding in which no colonic cause is found and an upper GI source has been ruled out, evaluation of the small bowel may be necessary.

REFERENCES AND SUGGESTED READINGS

Gostout GJ, Zuccaro G. A practical approach to acute lower gastrointestinal bleed. *Patient Care* 2000;29:23–31.

Peter DJ, Daugherty JM. Evaluation of the patient with gastrointestinal bleeding: an evidence based approach. *Emerg Med Clin North Am* 1999;17:239–261.

Yamada T. *Textbook and atlas of gastroenterology on CD-ROM.* Philadelphia: Lippincott Williams & Wilkins, 1999.

Zuccaro G Jr. Management of the adult patient with acute lower gastrointestinal bleeding. *Am J Gastroenterol* 1998;93:1202–1208.

Zuckerman GR, Prakash C. Acute lower intestinal bleeding part I: clinical presentation and diagnosis. *Gastrointest Endosc* 1998;48:606–616.

Zuckerman GR, Prakash C. Acute lower intestinal bleeding part II: etiology, therapy, and outcomes. *Gastrointest Endosc* 1999;49:228–238.

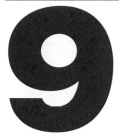

Occult Gastrointestinal Bleeding

Matthew H. Nissing

INTRODUCTION

Occult bleeding is defined as a positive fecal occult blood test (FOBT) without other evidence of blood in the stool. This bleeding may be continuous or intermittent and may cause an iron-deficiency anemia (IDA) depending on its chronicity and severity. It is the most common cause of IDA worldwide, especially in men and postmenopausal women.

CAUSES

Pathophysiology

Bleeding may occur from any portion of the GI tract. Depending on the location of the bleeding, hemoglobin may be absorbed, degraded, or excreted with feces. The globin chains of hemoglobin are degraded by proteases during transit. The heme moiety is cleaved from the globin and may be resorbed in the small intestine or modified by bacteria in the colon. Tests to measure occult blood are based on these properties.

IDA occurs when iron loss from occult bleeding depletes body iron stores. Occult bleeding and IDA probably represent a continuum of the same clinical spectrum; thus, the evaluations of the two conditions are very similar. The time to develop IDA depends on body stores of iron, rate of blood loss, and the ability of the body to increase iron absorption. Daily losses of approximately 10 mL are required to develop IDA. Iron deficiency is associated with fatigue, pica, achlorhydria, and a sprue-like small intestinal lesion causing malabsorption of fat and fat-soluble vitamins.

Differential Diagnosis

An extensive list of disorders may cause occult GI bleeding, with or without IDA. Table 9-1 lists the common causes of occult blood loss.

PRESENTATION

History and Physical Exam

By definition, there are no known symptoms of an occult GI bleed. However, it is important to question patients regarding diet, abdominal symptoms, and bowel movement history once a positive FOBT is found. Careful attention to medications, especially over-the-counter NSAIDs, is important. Symptoms that suggest IDA include fatigue, exertional dyspnea, tachycardia, and pica. Physical exam findings of IDA are rarely found in developed countries but may include brittle nails with longitudinal furrows or spooning (koilonychia), glossitis, cheilitis, and atrophic rhinitis. The Patterson-Kelly or Plummer-Vinson syndromes of postcricoid esophageal webs and IDA may occur. In absence of menorrhagia, gross hematuria, or obvious extraintestinal source, assume there is a GI source.

TABLE 9-1. SOURCES OF OCCULT GI BLEEDING

Source	Incidence (%)
Colorectal	25
Colorectal cancer	7
Polyps	9
Angiodysplasia	4
Colitis	1
Upper	41
Duodenal ulcer	5
Gastric ulcer	5
Esophagitis	11
Gastritis	8
Angiodysplasia	4
Gastric cancer	2
Celiac disease	1
No source found	41

MANAGEMENT
Fecal Occult Blood Tests

There are four basic types of FOBTs. Each has its own advantages and disadvantages. It is important to remember that a positive FOBT may not always indicate true disease. False-positive tests may occur due to diet, medications, or trauma while obtaining a sample. In fact, physiologic bleeding occurs in normal patients up to 1.5 mL/day.

- The radiochromium-labeled erythrocyte method is the accepted gold standard for quantifying GI blood loss, but it is not used clinically due to cost, complexity, and requirement of ≥ 3 days of stool collection.
- Guaiac (hemoccult) test is widely available, simple, and inexpensive. Guaiac is a colorless compound from tree bark that turns blue in the presence of peroxidase-like substances, such as heme and hydrogen peroxide. Therefore, guaiac tests detect free heme or heme bound to its apoprotein (e.g., globin, myoglobin, and certain cytochromes). They do not detect heme degradation products that may form with more proximal (upper GI) bleeding. Guaiac tests are not specific for blood and react with any peroxidase substance. False-positives occur from red meats or blood-containing foods as well as plant peroxidases, especially radishes. Iron does not cause false-positives. Vitamin C can cause a false-negative result.
- Immunochemical tests use antibodies against human hemoglobin. For this reason, they do not react with free heme and require no dietary restrictions. Some of these tests may be quantitative. However, because these tests detect globin, they are only useful for colorectal bleeding, as globin from gastric bleeding is degraded.
- Heme porphyrin assay (HemoQuant) is a quantitative fluorometric assay of heme and its degradation products. It has the advantage of detecting proximal bleeds, but it is a complex test requiring confirmation in a reference lab.

Diagnostic Evaluation

- Colonoscopy and esophagogastroduodenoscopy remain the primary means of investigating positive FOBT due to direct visualization of the mucosa and the ability to provide therapy during the procedure. Colonoscopy is typically performed first; if negative, then esophagogastroduodenoscopy is performed. These procedures are usually done during the same endoscopic session, thus eliminating the need for sedating the patient more than once.

• If comorbidities or patient preference preclude endoscopic evaluation, then barium enema and upper GI series can be substituted. These tests are limited by the inability to sample tissue or perform therapeutic intervention. Often, endoscopy is required after an abnormal radiographic study. Therefore, it is preferable to perform endoscopy as the initial test, if possible.

• If no etiology is identified after these studies, iron supplementation (oral or IV) should be initiated, with careful observation. If the anemia responds to iron supplementation and does not recur, then no further evaluation is required.

• If IDA persists despite oral iron supplementation or if FOBT remains persistently positive, then further evaluation is indicated. Repeat colonoscopy and esophagogastroduodenoscopy (or enteroscopy) should be performed initially, as lesions may have been missed on initial evaluation. If these tests are again negative, then the small bowel should be evaluated by enteroclysis, small bowel follow through, or enteroscopy (if not already done).

• At this point, the risks and benefits of further investigations need to be determined. Recently, capsule enteroscopy became available at some institutions for evaluation of the small bowel. This involves ingestion of a capsule containing a small camera that sends images to a recorder worn on the patient's belt. This method is still in the investigational phase, but it may prove to be useful if all other studies are negative. Other possible tests include angiography and intraop enteroscopy.

Treatment

Treatment is directed at the underlying problem. For those patients in whom no lesion can be identified, nonspecific therapy, such as iron supplementation and correction of coagulopathy/platelet disorders, is important.

KEY POINTS TO REMEMBER

• GI blood loss is the most common cause of IDA worldwide, especially in men and postmenopausal women.
• Occult bleeding and IDA probably represent a continuum of the same clinical spectrum; thus, the evaluations of the two conditions are very similar.
• Guaiac tests are the most commonly used FOBT. Given the intermittent bleeding of tumors and the sensitivity of the screening tests, any positive result requires investigation.
• Endoscopy is the primary mode of investigation.

REFERENCES AND SUGGESTED READINGS

Richter JM. Occult gastrointestinal bleeding. *Gastroenterol Clin North Am* 1994;23: 53–66.
Rockey DC, Cello JP. Evaluation of the gastrointestinal tract in patients with iron deficiency anemia. *N Engl J Med* 1993;329:1691–1695.
Rockey DC, Koch J, Cello JP, et al. Relative frequency of upper gastrointestinal and colonic lesions in patients with positive fecal occult blood tests. *N Engl J Med* 1998; 339:153–159.
Zuckerman G, Prakash C, Askin M, Lewis BS. AGA medical position statement: evaluation and management of occult and obscure gastrointestinal bleeding. *Gastroenterology* 2000;118:197–200.
Zuckerman G, Prakash C, Askin M, Lewis BS. AGA technical review on the evaluation and management of occult and obscure gastrointestinal bleeding. *Gastroenterology* 2000;118:201–221.

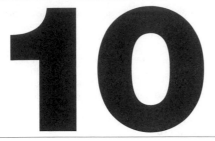

Jaundice

Aaron Shiels

INTRODUCTION

Jaundice is a common condition encountered in both inpatient and outpatient settings, with a broad spectrum of etiologies ranging from benign to life-threatening. Clinically, **jaundice** is defined as a yellow discoloration of skin, eyes, and mucous membranes caused by accumulation of bilirubin in body tissues. This typically becomes apparent when the serum bilirubin concentration reaches 2.5–3.0 mg/dL. Hyperbilirubinemia (serum bilirubin >1.5 mg/dL) may be present without overt jaundice, but it nevertheless represents an abnormal condition. Increased bilirubin levels may be due to a defect at any site along the bilirubin metabolic pathway, so an understanding of this pathway is essential in initiating the evaluation of a patient with jaundice.

CAUSES

Pathophysiology

Bilirubin is the end-product of heme breakdown (Fig. 10-1). Hemoglobin from senescent RBCs accounts for 80–90% of daily bilirubin. A smaller percentage comes from ineffective erythropoiesis and heme-containing proteins. Approximately 300 mg of bilirubin is produced daily. The reticuloendothelial system has the capacity to metabolize up to 1500 mg daily, so hemolysis rarely causes jaundice by itself, unless it is severe or associated with liver disease. Defects proximal to and including the conjugation step result in primarily unconjugated hyperbilirubinemia. Unconjugated or indirect hyperbilirubinemia is present when >80–85% of the total bilirubin is unconjugated. Defects after the glucuronidation step within the hepatocyte result in primarily conjugated hyperbilirubinemia. Conjugated or direct hyperbilirubinemia is present when >30% of the total bilirubin is in the conjugated form. Overlap between the two conditions may occur.

Differential Diagnosis

A defect at any step in bilirubin metabolism can result in hyperbilirubinemia and jaundice. This may be due to increased production of bilirubin, defective conjugation, hepatocellular dysfunction, impaired canalicular secretion, or biliary obstruction. Cases are divided into unconjugated and conjugated hyperbilirubinemia. The causes of each type are listed below.

Unconjugated Hyperbilirubinemia

1. Hemolysis and ineffective erythropoiesis: bilirubin usually <3–5 mg/dL, overt jaundice uncommon unless severe hemolysis or liver disease
2. Neonatal jaundice
3. Uridine diphosphate glucuronyl transferase deficiencies
   a. Gilbert's syndrome: autosomal-dominant transmission; affects 3–8% of population; presents with intermittent jaundice often precipitated by illness, stress, fatigue, or fasting; most common cause of hyperbilirubinemia in outpatients
   b. Crigler-Najjar types I and II

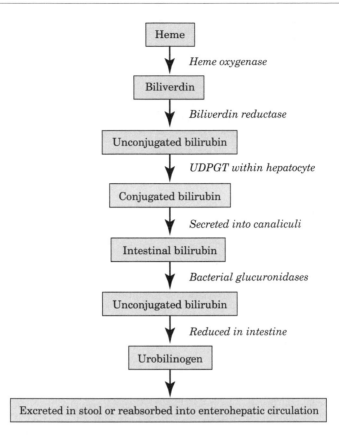

FIG. 10-1. Bilirubin metabolism. Heme oxygenase catalyzes the rate-limiting step within the reticuloendothelial system. Unconjugated bilirubin is transported bound primarily to albumin, at which point it is taken up by the hepatocyte and undergoes glucuronidation by uridine diphosphate glucuronyl transferase (UDPGT). It is then secreted in the water-soluble conjugated form into the canaliculi. Within the intestine, it is deconjugated and reduced by bacteria to urobilinogen, which is either excreted in stool or reabsorbed into the enterohepatic circulation. A defect at or before glucuronidation results in primarily unconjugated hyperbilirubinemia, whereas problems after this step cause conjugated hyperbilirubinemia.

4. Miscellaneous
   a. Resolving hematoma, hypothyroidism, thyrotoxicosis, fasting
   b. Drugs causing hemolysis: beta-lactams, isoniazid, quinine, quinidine, rifampin, sulfonamides, sulfonylureas, thiazides

Conjugated Hyperbilirubinemia

1. Congenital forms: Rotor syndrome, Dubin-Johnson syndrome, Byler disease
2. Familial forms: Benign recurrent intrahepatic cholestasis, cholestasis of pregnancy
3. Vascular causes: Hepatic vein thrombosis (Budd-Chiari syndrome), shock liver
4. Hepatocellular disorders
   a. Viral hepatitis, alcoholic liver disease, Wilson's disease, hemochromatosis, autoimmune hepatitis, alpha$_1$-antitrypsin deficiency

b. Drugs: acetaminophen, amiodarone, clindamycin, colchicine, ketoconazole, niacin, NSAIDs, salicylates, calcium channel blockers
5. Intrahepatic cholestasis
a. Infiltrative disorders: sarcoidosis, tumors, lymphoma, amyloid
b. Primary biliary cirrhosis
c. Infections: bacterial, sepsis, fungal, parasitic, AIDS
d. Postop
e. Stem cell transplant related: venoocclusive disease, graft-versus-host disease
f. Drugs: allopurinol, ampicillin, azathioprine, dapsone, erythromycin, estrogens, griseofulvin, haloperidol, hydralazine, nitrofurantoin, phenytoin, carbamazepine, zidovudine
6. Extrahepatic cholestasis
a. Gallstones
b. Strictures
c. Sclerosing cholangitis
d. Malignancies: pancreatic cancer, ampullary tumors
e. Chronic pancreatitis

PRESENTATION

The history, physical exam, and initial lab evaluation should be directed at answering the following questions:

• Is the hyperbilirubinemia unconjugated or conjugated?
• If unconjugated hyperbilirubinemia, is it due to increased production, decreased uptake, or impaired conjugation?
• If conjugated hyperbilirubinemia, is it due to intrahepatic or extrahepatic cholestasis?

History and Physical Exam

Aside from a thorough history and exam, the following specific points may help to identify the cause of the patient's jaundice. Patients <30 yrs are more likely to have acute parenchymal disease, whereas those >65 yrs are more likely to have gallstones or malignancy. In male patients, consider alcohol, pancreatic cancer, hepatocellular carcinoma, and hemochromatosis. In female patients, gallstones, primary biliary cirrhosis, and autoimmune hepatitis are more common. The presence of fever and right upper quadrant pain suggests cholangitis. Patients with viral hepatitis often give a history of viral prodrome, including anorexia, malaise, and myalgias. Infectious exposures, IV drug use, and prior blood transfusions also support the diagnosis of viral hepatitis. A careful alcohol and drug history, including over-the-counter and herbal remedies, is essential, as a multitude of drugs can cause jaundice (via hemolysis, hepatocellular damage, or intrahepatic cholestasis). Pruritus suggests a longer duration of disease and can be seen in both intrahepatic cholestasis and biliary obstruction.

The physical exam should focus on evidence of chronic liver disease, including muscle wasting, cachexia, palmar erythema, parotid enlargement, gynecomastia, and testicular atrophy. The findings of spider angiomata, palmar erythema, and caput medusae suggest cirrhosis. Ascites is usually seen in advanced cirrhosis but may also be seen with severe viral and alcoholic hepatitis. Asterixis and encephalopathy are nonspecific findings and suggest end-stage liver disease or fulminant hepatic failure. Other useful findings include a palpable abdominal mass, hyperpigmentation (hemochromatosis), xanthomas (primary biliary cirrhosis), and Kayser-Fleisher rings (Wilson's disease).

MANAGEMENT
Diagnostic Evaluation

Essential initial lab tests should include direct and indirect bilirubin, transaminases (AST and ALT), alkaline phosphatase, total protein, albumin, and PT. If lab results are consistent with **unconjugated hyperbilirubinemia,** then a hemolysis workup should be initiated. In the absence of hemolysis, most asymptomatic healthy patients with isolated unconjugated hyperbilirubinemia have Gilbert's disease and require no further evaluation. If lab results are consistent with conjugated hyperbilirubinemia or are indeterminate, then additional workup is required. Patients with transaminases elevated out of proportion to the alkaline phosphatase most likely have a hepatocellular disorder. If the alkaline phosphatase is elevated out of proportion to the transaminases, this suggests intrahepatic cholestasis or extrahepatic obstruction. An increased gamma-glutamyltransferase, 5'-nucleotidase, or leucine aminopeptidase confirms the hepatic origin of an elevated alkaline phosphatase. The presence of low albumin or prolonged PT suggests chronic liver disease with impaired synthetic function. However, prolonged PT may also be seen in obstructive jaundice. Of note, parenteral administration of vitamin K corrects the coagulopathy in patients with obstructive jaundice but not hepatocellular disease. Testing for urinary bilirubin or urobilinogen may be of some use, as clinical jaundice may lag behind bilirubinuria. Fig. 10-2 is helpful in planning the evaluation of the patient with jaundice.

The evaluation of **conjugated hyperbilirubinemia** requires careful selection of the appropriate imaging procedure, as many of these studies are expensive or invasive. If the initial evaluation suggests a possible vascular cause (Budd-Chiari or shock liver), then U/S with Doppler should be the initial study to evaluate patency of the hepatic and portal veins and hepatic artery. Increased transaminases should prompt a search for hepatocellular disorders. If the history and exam cause concern for malignancy, then an abdominal CT scan and AFP should be ordered, followed by U/S- or CT-guided liver biopsy, if appropriate. If the initial evaluation does not reveal an obvious etiology (alcohol, drugs, infections), then specific biochemical studies should be ordered, including viral hepatitis serologies, ANA, antimitochondrial antibody, immunoglobulins, iron studies, ceruloplasmin, and alpha$_1$-antitrypsin levels. If the cause still remains unclear, then liver biopsy should be considered. Patients with increased alkaline phosphatase should be evaluated for causes of cholestatic jaundice. U/S should be the initial study to evaluate for evidence of biliary ductal dilatation. Abdominal CT can also be used to evaluate for ductal dilatation, but it has specific limitations (see below for discussion of advantages and disadvantages of the various imaging procedures). If ductal dilatation is present, or if the suspicion for obstruction remains high despite a normal study, then endoscopic retrograde cholangiopancreatography (ERCP) or percutaneous transhepatic cholangiography (PTC) (see below) should be performed. Of note, patients who have undergone prior cholecystectomy normally have a dilated common bile duct. If ductal dilatation is not seen and the suspicion for obstruction is low, then biochemical studies should be ordered as above to look for parenchymal disease. Again, liver biopsy should be considered if no etiology can be identified.

Imaging Procedures

Ultrasound
U/S is the best initial study for detection of biliary obstruction as evidenced by ductal dilatation. Of note, biliary obstruction cannot be ruled out definitively by nondilated ducts. Therefore, additional studies are required if a high suspicion of obstruction remains. U/S can also identify hepatic parenchymal lesions, gallbladder disease, cholelithiasis, and choledocholithiasis. Its advantages are portability, noninvasiveness, and relatively low cost. Disadvantages include operator-dependent nature and decreased image quality in obese patients or those with overlying bowel gas.

Abdominal CT
Abdominal CT is a first-line study for evaluation of hepatic parenchymal lesions; it is also an alternative to U/S for identifying biliary obstruction. Its advantages are its less operator-dependent nature and improved images in obese patients. Limitations include higher cost, lack of portability, inability to detect noncalcified gallstones, and requirement of radiocontrast dye.

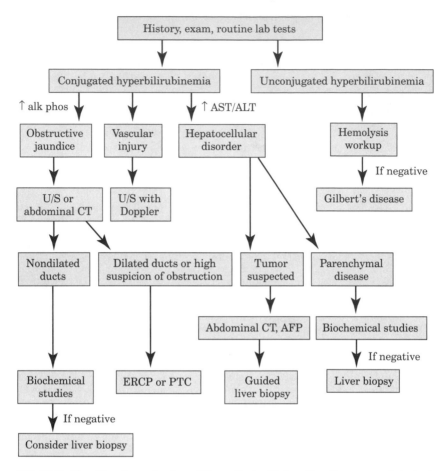

FIG. 10-2. Algorithm for evaluation of the patient with jaundice. See comments in text regarding selection of appropriate imaging study when given a choice in the algorithm. alk phos, alkaline phosphatase; ERCP, endoscopic retrograde cholangiopancreatography; PTC, percutaneous transhepatic cholangiography.

Endoscopic Retrograde Cholangiopancreatography

ERCP is an excellent test for evaluation of biliary obstruction because it provides direct visualization of the biliary and pancreatic ducts. Advantages include high accuracy in locating the site of obstruction as well as ability to perform therapeutic interventions (sphincterotomy, stone extraction, stent placement). Disadvantages include expense, invasiveness, difficulty after certain surgeries (Roux-en-Y), and morbidity. Complications of perforation, bleeding, cholangitis, and pancreatitis are uncommon but can be serious.

Magnetic Resonance Cholangiopancreatography

Magnetic resonance cholangiopancreatography is a useful test for assessing liver parenchyma and biliary tract. Advantages include its noninvasive nature and ability to accurately identify various liver lesions. Unlike ERCP, it does not have therapeutic capabilities.

Percutaneous Transhepatic Cholangiography

PTC is also a good test for evaluation of biliary obstruction, with accuracy similar to ERCP in identifying the site of biliary obstruction if the ducts are dilated. However, it is less accurate than ERCP if there are nondilated ducts, and several passes into the liver may be required to access the biliary tree. Advantages include lower cost and therapeutic capabilities (decompression of biliary system). Aside from limited usefulness with nondilated ducts, other problems include inability to perform in the presence of coagulopathy and ascites as well as complication risks (bleeding, sepsis, pneumothorax, peritonitis). The decision of whether to perform ERCP or PTC should be based partially on local expertise of the gastroenterologists and radiologists.

KEY POINTS TO REMEMBER

- Unconjugated or indirect hyperbilirubinemia is usually defined as >80–85% of the total bilirubin in the unconjugated form.
- Conjugated or direct hyperbilirubinemia is present when >30% of the total bilirubin is in the conjugated form.
- Hemolysis usually presents with bilirubin levels <3–5 mg/dL, and overt jaundice is uncommon unless there is severe hemolysis or concomitant liver disease.
- In the absence of hemolysis, most asymptomatic healthy patients with isolated unconjugated hyperbilirubinemia have Gilbert's disease and require no further evaluation.
- Patients with transaminases elevated out of proportion to the alkaline phosphatase most likely have a hepatocellular disorder.
- If the alkaline phosphatase is elevated out of proportion to the transaminases, this suggests intrahepatic cholestasis or extrahepatic obstruction.
- If U/S demonstrates dilated ducts, or if the clinical suspicion for obstruction remains high despite a normal U/S, then ERCP or PTC should be performed.

REFERENCES AND SUGGESTED READINGS

Bacon BR, DiBisceglie AM. *Liver disease: diagnosis and management.* New York: Churchill Livingstone, 2000:36–46.

Berk PD, Noyer D. Bilirubin and hyperbilirubinemia. *Semin Liver Dis* 1994:14;325–355.

Green RM, Flamm S. AGA technical review on the evaluation of liver chemistry tests. *Gastroenterology* 2002:123;1367–1384.

Sleisenger MH, Fordtran JS. *Gastrointestinal disease: pathophysiology, diagnosis, management,* 5th ed. Philadelphia: WB Saunders, 1993:1765–1776.

Tiribelli C, Ostrow JD. New concepts in bilirubin and jaundice: report of the Third International Bilirubin Workshop, April 6–8, 1995, Trieste, Italy. *Hepatology* 1996; 24:1296–1311.

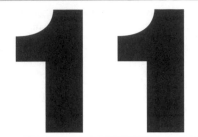

Abnormal Liver Chemistries

John T. Battaile

INTRODUCTION

The evaluation of a patient with suspected hepatic or biliary disease can be aided by the measurement of various serum markers of liver function or injury. A thorough understanding of these markers of hepatic disease is essential for proper interpretation and accurate diagnosis. Whereas a single lab value rarely leads to a diagnosis in patients with hepatic disease, the pattern of liver enzyme abnormalities together with a thorough history and physical exam can help to direct additional workup to arrive at a diagnosis.

SERUM ENZYMES

Aminotransferases

AST (SGOT) and ALT (SGPT) are sensitive markers of hepatocellular injury or necrosis. ALT is the more specific indicator of liver injury because it is found primarily in the liver, whereas AST can be found in liver, cardiac and skeletal muscle, kidney, brain, pancreas, and other sites. A nonhepatic source should be considered in isolated elevations of AST. Marked elevations in AST and ALT (often >1000 U/L) are seen in acute viral, toxin-induced, and ischemic hepatitis. Small to moderate elevations in the transaminases are seen in a number of conditions, including chronic viral hepatitis, alcohol abuse, autoimmune hepatitis, nonalcoholic fatty liver disease, biliary obstruction, hemochromatosis, Wilson's disease, and alpha$_1$-antitrypsin deficiency, and as a side effect of various medicines (Table 11-1). The pattern of elevation can offer clues as to etiology. An AST:ALT ratio of ≥ 2 is highly suggestive of alcohol-induced injury, whereas a ratio of <1 is usually seen in patients with acute or chronic viral hepatitis or extrahepatic biliary obstruction.

Alkaline Phosphatase

Elevated alkaline phosphatase (AP) levels arise from two main sources—liver and bone—but the enzyme is also found in other tissues, including placenta, which explains the elevations in AP among women in the third trimester of pregnancy. Elevations in AP are seen in a variety of hepatobiliary conditions, including cholestatic syndromes (e.g., biliary obstruction, primary biliary cirrhosis, primary sclerosing cholangitis, and drug-induced cholestasis). It is also elevated in infiltrative processes (sarcoidosis, other granulomatous diseases), liver metastasis, and, to a lesser extent, any form of liver disease. Elevations in AP can be confirmed as hepatic in origin by measuring either gamma-glutamyltransferase (GGT) or 5'-nucleotidase.

Gamma-Glutamyltransferase

GGT is found in bile duct epithelial cells, hepatocytes, and other tissues, including kidney, pancreas, and intestine. In the evaluation of hepatobiliary disease, it has two

TABLE 11-1. DRUGS COMMONLY ASSOCIATED WITH ELEVATED LIVER ENZYMES

Antiarrhythmics	Analgesics
Amiodarone	Acetaminophen
Antibiotics	NSAIDs
Synthetic penicillins	Sulfonylureas
Ciprofloxacin	Glipizide
Nitrofurantoin	Homeopathic substances
Ketoconazole	Ephedra
Fluconazole	Ji bu huan
Isoniazid	Senna
Erythromycin	Chaparral
Antihypertensives	Drugs of abuse
Methyldopa	Anabolic steroids
Captopril	Cocaine
Enalapril	3,4-Methylelenedioxy-methamphet-
Antiepileptics	amine ("ecstasy")
Phenytoin	Phencyclidine
Carbamazepine	Toluene-containing glues
Hydroxymethylglutaryl coenzyme A	Chloroform
reductase inhibitors	Trichloroethylene
Atorvastatin	
Pravastatin	
Lovastatin	
Simvastatin	

main uses. An elevated level helps confirm hepatobiliary origin of elevated AP. GGT also serves as a useful tool in diagnosing chronic alcohol abuse. A GGT that is twice the normal level in a patient with an AST:ALT ratio >2 is highly suggestive of alcohol abuse. The utility of GGT is somewhat limited by its lack of specificity. Elevations in GGT can be seen in a number of disorders, including pancreatic diseases, myocardial infarction, COPD, renal failure, diabetes, and rheumatoid arthritis, as well as with the use of phenytoin, warfarin, barbiturates, and other drugs that induce microsomal enzymes.

5'-Nucleotidase

Like GGT, 5'-nucleotidase can be used to confirm hepatic origin of elevated AP.

EXCRETORY PRODUCTS

Bilirubin

Bilirubin is a degradation product of hemoglobin and hemoproteins composed of conjugated (direct) and unconjugated (indirect) fractions. Unconjugated hyperbilirubinemia results from excessive production, reduced hepatic uptake, or impaired conjugation of bilirubin. Conjugated hyperbilirubinemia occurs as a result of impaired intrahepatic secretion of bilirubin or extrahepatic biliary obstruction. Both forms of hyperbilirubinemia manifest clinically as jaundice. A complete discussion of the pathophysiology and differential diagnosis of jaundice is in Chap. 10, Jaundice.

Serum Bile Acids

Cholic acid and chenodeoxycholic acid are synthesized from cholesterol in the liver and converted by bacteria in the intestine to deoxycholic and lithocholic acid, the secondary bile acids. Elevated levels of serum bile acids are specific markers of liver disease; however, the sensitivity is low, especially in mild disease, limiting their clinical utility.

MEASURES OF SYNTHETIC FUNCTION

Clotting Factors

Many of the proteins involved in hemostasis, including the coagulation factors, are synthesized in the liver. Normal activity of clotting factors II, VII, IX, and X depends on normal hepatic synthetic function as well as the presence of vitamin K. As a result, two forms of hepatobiliary dysfunction can lead to coagulopathy manifested by pro-longation of PT.

- Significant hepatocellular injury or necrosis can impair hepatic synthetic function of clotting factors and leads to PT prolongation.
- Cholestatic syndromes may also prolong PT by interfering with intestinal absorption of vitamin K via impaired lipid absorption. This form should respond to parenteral administration of vitamin K, whereas coagulopathy purely from impaired hepatic synthesis should not.

Albumin

Serum albumin concentration is often decreased in chronic liver disease and reflects decreased synthesis. Other disease states as well as plasma volume expansion can also decrease albumin concentration. Levels may be normal in acute liver disease due to a half-life of approximately 20 days.

DIAGNOSTIC EVALUATION

A series of lab tests alone rarely leads to a diagnosis in a patient suspected of having hepatobiliary disease. Instead, the clinical context must be considered, and carefully chosen disease-specific lab tests and other appropriate studies are necessary to arrive at a diagnosis. A thorough and accurate history is essential in the approach to a patient with abnormal liver chemistries; it should include the following:

- Symptoms of liver disease (e.g., weight loss, anorexia, fever, nausea, vomiting, abdominal pain, pruritus, jaundice).
- Medical and surgical history.
- Careful review of prescription and over-the-counter medications.
- Thorough social history, including history of alcohol consumption, illicit drug use, use of herbal remedies, sick contacts and exposure history, well water consumption, tattoos, recent travel, dietary history, sexual and menstrual history, occupational and environmental history, and transfusion history.
- Family history of jaundice may be present in Gilbert syndrome, Dubin-Johnson, and hereditary hemolytic syndromes. Hemochromatosis, Wilson's disease, and alpha$_1$-antitrypsin deficiency are autosomal-recessive disorders. Other hepatobiliary disorders, including primary sclerosing cholangitis, primary biliary cirrhosis, and autoimmune hepatitis, may also have a genetic component.

The physical exam should focus on stigmata of liver disease as well as signs suggestive of systemic diseases that commonly affect the liver.

A nonhepatic source must be considered in any patient with abnormal liver chemistries. When a **hepatic source** is suspected, it is helpful to divide the pattern of abnormality into one of three broad categories: *hepatocellular injury, cholestasis,* and *infiltrative processes.*

Hepatocellular Injury

Hepatocellular injury typically manifests with modest to profound elevations in serum aminotransferases. AP and bilirubin may or may not be elevated depending on the nature and severity of the injury. As a general rule, the highest elevations in transaminases are seen with ischemic and acute viral hepatitis. (See also Chap. 20, Acute Liver Disease). Toxic injury is also typically associated with marked elevations in AST and ALT. Less-marked elevations in transaminases are seen with chronic viral hepatitis and cirrhosis. PT can be prolonged with hepatocellular injury depending on the extent of hepatocellular necrosis and subsequent hepatic synthetic dysfunction. Albumin is normal in acute injury but may decrease in chronic disorders when synthetic function is significantly impaired. Table 11-2 lists the common causes of hepatocellular injuries. The initial evaluation should include specific testing of the most likely etiologies. Specific biochemical testing often reveals the etiology. Imaging with U/S or abdominal CT may be useful in identifying structural causes. For patients with unexplained abnormal transaminases, liver biopsy should be considered, especially if the levels remain elevated for >6 mos.

Cholestasis

Cholestatic injury typically produces moderate to profound elevations in AP often with hyperbilirubinemia (elevations in bilirubin may be absent in certain clinical situations, such as with partial biliary obstruction). PT may be prolonged but responds to parenteral vitamin K administration. Depending on the nature of the cholestasis, serum transaminases may or may not be elevated. In early total common bile duct obstruction, AST and ALT may rise before AP. Evaluating a patient with cholestatic injury by routine liver chemistries can be particularly challenging. Once a nonhepatic source of elevated AP has been excluded, selection of other studies is directed by the degree of AP elevation. Table 11-3 lists the common causes of cholestasis. U/S is the

TABLE 11-2. CAUSES OF HEPATOCELLULAR INJURY PATTERN OF LIVER CHEMISTRIES

Viral hepatitis (A, B, C, D, E, CMV, Epstein-Barr virus, herpes simplex virus, VZV)

Cirrhosis

Alcoholic liver disease

Nonalcoholic fatty liver disease

Wilson's disease

Hemochromatosis

Shock liver (hypotension)

Budd-Chiari syndrome

Venoocclusive disease

Acute fatty liver of pregnancy

Autoimmune hepatitis

Alpha$_1$-antitrypin deficiency

Medications

CMV, cytomegalovirus; VZV, varicella-zoster virus.

TABLE 11-3. CAUSES OF CHOLESTATIC INJURY PATTERN OF LIVER CHEMISTRIES

Malignancy (intrahepatic or extrahepatic)
Biliary stricture
Choledocholithiasis
Primary sclerosing cholangitis
Primary biliary cirrhosis
Sepsis
Rotor's or Dubin-Johnson syndrome
Medications

best initial study, as it allows visualization of the liver parenchyma and biliary tree. Depending on the U/S findings, further evaluation may include abdominal CT, endoscopic retrograde cholangiopancreatography, or liver biopsy.

Infiltrative Process

Infiltrative liver injury is seen most commonly with granulomatous diseases, including sarcoidosis and metastatic disease to the liver. The predominant feature is an elevation in AP and, to a lesser extent, elevated bilirubin. Unlike with cholestatic liver injury, PT prolongation would not be expected in infiltrative injury because intestinal absorption of vitamin K is not affected. Table 11-4 lists the common causes of infiltrative liver disease. Imaging with either U/S or abdominal CT, often followed by liver biopsy, forms the basis for evaluating infiltrative processes.

KEY POINTS TO REMEMBER

• ALT is the more specific indicator of liver injury because it is found primarily in the liver, whereas AST can be found in liver, cardiac and skeletal muscle, kidney, brain, pancreas, and other sites.
• Marked elevations in AST and ALT (often >1000 U/L) are seen in acute viral, toxin-induced, and ischemic hepatitis.
• Elevations in AP can be confirmed as hepatic in origin by measuring either GGT or 5'-nucleotidase.
• Cholestatic syndromes may prolong PT by interfering with intestinal absorption of vitamin K via impaired lipid absorption. This form should respond to parenteral administration of vitamin K, whereas coagulopathy purely from impaired hepatic synthesis should not.
• For patients with unexplained abnormal chemistries, liver biopsy should be considered, especially if the levels remain elevated for >6 mos.
• Imaging with either U/S or abdominal CT, often followed by liver biopsy, forms the basis for evaluating infiltrative processes.

TABLE 11-4. CAUSES OF INFILTRATIVE INJURY PATTERN OF LIVER CHEMISTRIES

Metastatic cancer	Tuberculosis
Lymphoma	Sarcoidosis
Leukemia	Histoplasmosis
Primary hepatic tumors	Medications

REFERENCES AND SUGGESTED READINGS

Green RM, Flamm S. AGA technical review on the evaluation of liver chemistry tests. *Gastroenterology* 2002:123;1367–1384.

Moselely R. Approach to the patient with abnormal liver chemistries. In: Yamada T, ed. *Textbook of gastroenterology*. Philadelphia: Lippincott Williams & Wilkins, 1999.

Moseley R. Evaluation of abnormal liver chemistry tests. *Med Clin North Am* 1996; 80:887–906.

Pratt D, Kaplan M. Evaluation of abnormal liver-enzyme results in asymptomatic patients. *N Engl J Med* 2000;342(17):1266–1271.

Pratt D, Kaplan M. Laboratory tests. In: Schiff E, Sorrell M, Maddrey W, eds. *Schiff's diseases of the liver*, 8th ed. Vol. 1. Philadelphia: Lippincott–Raven, 1999:205–244.

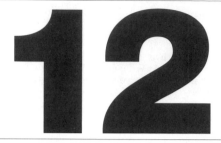

Ascites

Clinton T. Snedegar

INTRODUCTION

Ascites is the abnormal accumulation of fluid in the peritoneal cavity. The causes of ascites are myriad, but the most common cause by far is portal HTN secondary to cirrhosis of the liver. Once ascites develops in a patient with end-stage liver disease, the 1-yr survival drops by as much as 50%. The presence of ascites can also lead to spontaneous bacterial peritonitis (SBP), hepatorenal syndrome, and hepatic hydrothorax. Development of ascites is one criterion used in determining the need for liver transplantation.

CAUSES

Liver Disease

As a result of altered hepatic architecture, sinusoidal pressure increases in the fibrotic liver. This increase leads to increased hydrostatic pressure in the liver and splanchnic bed and accumulation of fluid in the peritoneum. Cirrhosis also causes peripheral vasodilation, probably secondary to increased levels of arterial nitric oxide. This vasodilatory effect yields an effectively reduced plasma volume, initiating renal protective mechanisms and the renin-angiotensin-aldosterone system. The kidney avidly retains sodium and water, furthering fluid accumulation in a vicious cycle.

Malignancy

Tumors may lead to ascites in several ways. In peritoneal carcinomatosis, proteinaceous material exuded into the peritoneal cavity produces an osmotic gradient with movement of fluid from the intravascular space. Hepatocellular carcinoma can cause portal HTN via replacement of normal liver parenchyma. Carcinoma-induced hypercoagulable states can cause hepatic or portal venous thrombosis with subsequent ascites.

Cardiac Disease

Ascites due to heart failure is fairly uncommon. The fluid accumulation likely results from circulatory compromise and activation of antinatriuretic, renin-angiotensin, and sympathetic nervous systems. Constrictive pericarditis, on the other hand, commonly causes ascites.

Infections

Peritoneal TB leads to proteinaceous exudate and subsequent movement of fluid into the peritoneal cavity.

Acute Pancreatitis

Pancreatic ascites results from a pancreatic enzyme leak in severe acute pancreatitis. This can cause an intraperitoneal chemical burn yielding further problems.

Chylous Ascites

Obstruction of the thoracic duct may be seen with lymphoma or surgical trauma.

Nephrotic Syndrome

Patients with nephrotic syndrome have anasarca in addition to ascites, and ascites is furthered via activation of renal protective mechanisms.

SLE

Serositis may yield an inflammatory ascites in the connective tissue disorder of SLE.

PRESENTATION

History and Physical Exam

A thorough history and physical exam are essential, particularly in patients with new-onset ascites. The patient with ascites usually develops increased abdominal girth, often manifest as weight gain or increase in belt size. Ascites is usually not painful except in cases complicated by peritonitis, but tense ascites may be very uncomfortable. Physical exam may reveal bulging flanks, shifting dullness, or the presence of a fluid wave. These signs are usually present if $\geq$ 500 cc of fluid are present. U/S exam of the abdomen may be helpful if the diagnosis is in doubt. Other physical signs may be helpful in identifying specific causes of ascites (e.g., jaundice, palmar erythema, and spider angiomata in chronic liver disease; jugular venous distention and an audible S_3 in congestive heart failure).

MANAGEMENT

Diagnostic Evaluation

A diagnostic paracentesis should be performed in all patients with new-onset ascites or in any patient with known ascites and abdominal pain, fever, leukocytosis, decompensation of liver disease, or other illness requiring hospitalization. Fluid should be obtained in a sterile fashion and evaluated for automated cell count and differential, albumin, protein, lactic dehydrogenase, glucose, and culture. The sensitivity of ascites fluid culture is increased if the culture bottles are inoculated at the bedside. If the clinical situation suggests other less common causes, fluid may also be sent for amylase and triglyceride levels, cytology, flow cytometry, or mycobacterial smear and culture.

The most important item in stratifying the diagnostic workup is the **serum-ascites albumin gradient (SAAG)**, which is simply the number obtained by subtracting the ascites albumin level from the serum albumin level in g/dL. The values for albumin from serum and ascites fluid should be obtained at a relatively close interval, preferably the same day. A SAAG of $\geq$ 1.1 g/dL is indicative of portal HTN–related ascites with 97% specificity.

Obtaining the cell count and differential is the most efficient way to determine if the ascitic fluid is infected. A neutrophil count of >250 cells/μL or total WBC count of >500 cells/μL is the cutoff used for diagnosis of SBP and initiation of empiric antibiotic therapy.

An ascitic protein level of <1.0 g/dL places a patient in a high-risk group for SBP. In patients with secondarily infected ascites (e.g., from GI tract perforation), ascitic protein and lactic dehydrogenase are high, and the glucose level is low. Secondarily infected ascites often requires surgical intervention.

Amylase levels are helpful in detecting pancreatic ascites, and triglyceride levels help identify chylous ascites. Cytology is useful when peritoneal carcinomatosis is suspected but is less likely to be positive in hepatocellular carcinoma. If the cell count is remarkable for a high number of lymphocytes, TB or lymphoma is suspected. AFB stain and culture or flow cytometry can confirm the diagnosis.

Treatment

Treatment of ascites depends on the etiology. For example, the same management techniques for ascites associated with liver disease are appropriate for malignancy. For the purposes of this chapter, we limit discussion to ascites in chronic liver disease.

Management of ascites in cirrhosis should be initiated in a stepwise fashion based on response to the specific interventions discussed below.

Sodium Restriction

Management should begin with sodium restriction to 2 g/day. Although this may be insufficient in many cases, it is nearly impossible for patients to adhere to a stricter regimen in a nonhospital setting. Patients should be cautioned to avoid salt supplements containing potassium chloride, as use of these products can lead to life-threatening hyperkalemia, especially in association with aldosterone antagonists. Fluid restriction is usually not necessary but should be initiated in patients with dilutional hyponatremia (serum sodium <125 mmol/L).

Diuretic Therapy

Diuretic therapy is a necessary addition to dietary sodium restriction in most cases. The goal of diuretic therapy should be a daily weight loss of 1 kg in patients with edema and 0.5 kg without edema until ascites is adequately controlled. The diuretic can then be adjusted for maintenance. Because increased sodium uptake in the distal convoluted tubule under the influence of aldosterone is the predominant mechanism of sodium retention in cirrhosis, initiation of spironolactone is the best choice for initial therapy. Spironolactone, 100 mg/day, in a single oral dose is recommended for initiation. The dose can be increased by 100 mg every 1–2 wks until the maximum dose of 400 mg/day is achieved or significant side effects occur. Common side effects include hyperkalemia and gynecomastia. If patients are unable to tolerate spironolactone in therapeutic doses due to gynecomastia, amiloride or triamterene may also be used, although these are less effective agents for controlling ascites. Patients who do not achieve effective diuresis with spironolactone alone should be started on a loop diuretic, such as furosemide, 40 mg/day, once the dose of spironolactone has reached 200 mg/day. It is important to note that with the initiation of loop diuretics, patients must be carefully observed for signs of intravascular volume depletion, renal insufficiency, and decompensation of liver disease. Furosemide alone is not adequate therapy in cirrhotic ascites. No diuretic therapy should be initiated in a patient with an unstable creatinine due to the risk of precipitating the hepatorenal syndrome.

Large Volume Paracentesis

At one time, large volume paracentesis (LVP) was the only reasonable therapy for ascites. Today, LVP remains an excellent technique to provide relief from the discomfort of tense ascites. Rare but important complications of LVP are cardiovascular collapse and renal failure. Some studies indicate that infusion of albumin (5–8 g albumin/L ascites removed) minimizes the likelihood of these complications and should be considered in high-risk patients or those with LVP of >5 L.

Transjugular Intrahepatic Portosystemic Shunting

Transjugular intrahepatic portosystemic shunting is currently the most effective method of managing ascites refractory to diuretic use. The goal of this procedure is to lower portal pressures by providing a shunt from the portal vein through the liver directly to the hepatic vein. This is achieved by accessing the hepatic vein via a jugular approach, puncturing liver tissue to access an intrahepatic portal vein, and establishing a conduit via an expandable stent. Major complications include hepatic encephalopathy and decompensated cirrhosis. These complications are more likely to occur in Child-Turcotte-Pugh class C liver disease.

KEY POINTS TO REMEMBER

- In cirrhosis, ascites formation is related not only to a hydrostatic pressure gradient, but also to decreased effective plasma volume secondary to peripheral vasodilation and subsequent sodium and water retention by the kidney in response to the renin-angiotensin-aldosterone system.

- Diagnostic paracentesis should be performed on all patients with new-onset ascites and in those with established ascites and new symptoms or decompensation of liver disease.
- The SAAG is the most important determinant in the diagnostic evaluation of new-onset ascites. An SAAG of ≥ 1.1 g/dL is very specific for portal HTN–related ascites.
- Ascitic neutrophil count of >250 cells/μL or total WBC count of >500 cells/μL is indicative of SBP and should prompt initiation of empiric antibiotic therapy.
- Management of ascites in cirrhosis should advance in a stepwise fashion with dietary sodium restriction, incremental addition of spironolactone and loop diuretics, and LVP in cases of tense ascites.
- Transjugular intrahepatic portosystemic shunting is currently the most effective therapy for refractory ascites, but it carries a significant risk of precipitating encephalopathy or liver decompensation.

REFERENCES AND SUGGESTED READINGS

Garcia-Tsao G. Current management of the complications of cirrhosis and portal hypertension. *Gastroenterology* 2001;120:726–748.

Lake J. The role of transjugular portosystemic shunting in patients with ascites. *N Engl J Med* 2000;342:1745–1747.

Runyon B. Approach to the patient with ascites. In: Yamada T, ed. *Textbook and atlas of gastroenterology on CD-ROM*. Philadelphia: Lippincott Williams & Wilkins, 1999.

Runyon B. Care of patients with ascites. *N Engl J Med* 1994;330:337–342.

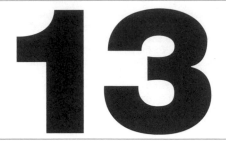

Nutrition

Patrick B. McDonough

INTRODUCTION

Assessment of nutritional status is an important aspect of the care of all patients. At present, there is no gold standard for evaluating the nutritional status of hospitalized patients. The best overall approach involves a thorough clinical and physical exam, a nutritional history, and appropriate lab studies.

FUNCTIONAL ASSESSMENT

Functional assessment includes identification of preexisting malnutrition before acute presentation, relevant medical and surgical history, medications, social habits, and a focused dietary history. The presence of mild (<5%), moderate (5–10%), or severe (>10%) unintentional weight loss in the last 6 mos should be determined. Unintentional weight loss of >10% is associated with a poor clinical outcome. Physical exam should include careful inspection of hair, skin, eyes, mouth, extremities, and fluid status as stigmata for protein calorie malnutrition or vitamin and mineral deficiencies. Temporal muscle wasting, sunken supraclavicular fossae, and decreased adipose stores are easily recognized signs of starvation. Malnutrition may be related to dysfunction of cardiovascular, respiratory, and GI systems. BMI is a useful indicator of nutritional status (Table 13-1).

METABOLIC ASSESSMENT

Most lab measures of nutritional status have poor sensitivity and specificity. A thorough history and physical exam provide much more useful information. However, there are some parameters that deserve mention.

Serum Albumin

A serum albumin value of <2.2 g/dL generally reflects severe malnutrition. However, the reliability of albumin as a marker of visceral protein status is compromised by its long half-life of 14–20 days, making it less responsive to acute changes in nutritional status. In addition, albumin is decreased in conditions other than malnutrition, including any acute illness, liver disease, nephrotic syndrome, and protein-losing enteropathy.

Prealbumin

Prealbumin is a more reliable indicator due to a shorter half-life of 24–48 hrs. It is more indicative of a patient's current nutritional state. However, as is the case with albumin, its concentration is diminished by renal and liver disease.

Transferrin

Transferrin has a half-life of 9 days, with intermediate sensitivity for incipient malnutrition.

TABLE 13-1. BODY MASS INDEX (BMI)

BMI = weight in kg/(height in m)^2

<18.5	Underweight
18.5–24.9	Normal
25–29.9	Overweight
30–34.9	Class I obesity
35–39.9	Class II obesity
>40	Class III obesity

Lymphocyte Count

Compromise of cell-mediated immunity due to malnutrition is suggested by a total lymphocyte count <1000/mm^3 or a lack of skin test induration >5 mm through delayed hypersensitivity testing with glycerin control at 48 hrs. This is also a nonspecific test.

MALNUTRITION

Malnutrition causes a number of deleterious side effects:

- Increased susceptibility to infection
- Poor wound healing
- Increased frequency of decubitus ulcers
- Overgrowth of bacteria in the GI tract
- Abnormal nutrient losses though the stool

A 30-day mortality rate of 62% was seen among patients whose plasma albumin was <2 mg/dL. Metabolic derangements are amplified during periods of critical illness, and protein calorie malnutrition is particularly detrimental in this situation. Patients most likely to benefit from nutritional support are those with baseline malnutrition in whom a protracted period of starvation would otherwise occur.

NUTRITIONAL SUPPORT

There are no absolute indications for nutritional support, either enteral or parenteral. A careful assessment of the patient's clinical condition and expected outcome helps to determine the need for nutritional support. The amount of time that a patient can tolerate inadequate nutrition varies considerably and is often difficult to quantify precisely. Factors that must be accounted for include amount of intake, amount of available endogenous stores (adipose tissue), lean muscle mass, and the rate of catabolism. Individuals who are severely malnourished at the outset of an illness often need nutritional support immediately, whereas patients with adequate stores can tolerate longer periods without adequate nutritional intake. The decision to initiate nutritional support must be individualized and the type of support carefully chosen. The two general types of nutritional support are enteral and parenteral.

Enteral Nutrition

The most important rule regarding nutritional support is summarized as follows: "If the gut works, use it." Enteral feeding is considered cheaper, safer, and more physiologic in that it preserves GI tract barrier function. Mechanical obstruction is the only absolute contraindication to enteral feedings. Other relative contraindications include ileus, GI bleeding, severe pancreatitis, and enteric fistulas. There are some general principles to consider when initiating enteral nutritional support.

- For short-term support (<30 days), NG or nasoenteric tubes are preferred over gastrostomy or jejunostomy tubes.

- Tubes placed past the third portion of the duodenum, and especially past the ligament of Treitz, are associated with a decreased risk of aspiration.
- Prokinetic drugs given before placement may be beneficial in positioning smaller nasoenteric tubes (8–10 French) beyond the pylorus.
- Intermittent gravity feeding is sufficient for most patients with NG or gastrostomy tubes. Pump-controlled infusions are recommended for jejunal feedings to decrease bloating, abdominal discomfort, and diarrhea.
- With NG tube feeding, a single elevated residual volume is an indication to recheck the residual volume in 1 hr. However, the feeding should not automatically be stopped.
- Jejunal access is appropriate in patients with a history of tube feeding–related aspiration pneumonia or severe reflux esophagitis.
- Gastrostomy tubes are indicated if the duration of enteral feeding is expected to be >30 days. The underlying condition and local expertise should dictate percutaneous, radiologic, or surgically placed gastrostomy tubes.

Complications of Tube Feedings

Tube feeding is a relatively safe procedure, and complications usually can be avoided or adequately managed. In addition to the complications of percutaneous tube placement (infection, bleeding, inadvertent colonic placement), patients may experience aspiration, diarrhea, and alterations in drug absorption and metabolism.

To limit the risk of aspiration, the head of the patient's bed should be raised ≥ 45 degrees during feeding and for 1 hr afterward. Intermittent or continuous feeding regimens, rather than the rapid bolus method, should be used. Gastric residuals should be checked regularly, and all patients should be observed for signs of feeding intolerance.

Jejunal access is helpful in patients with recurrent tube feeding aspiration (not oropharyngeal) or in critically ill patients at risk for impaired gastric motility. Severe vomiting or coughing may displace some nonsurgical tubes, and radiographs may be needed to verify tube position.

Parenteral Nutrition

Parenteral nutrition should be given if the GI tract is not accessible or functional, as occurs in patients with bowel obstruction, ileus, necrotizing enterocolitis, severe pancreatitis, diffuse peritonitis, intractable vomiting, or short gut syndrome. Hypotension with hemodynamic instability is associated with reduced intestinal blood flow, and low tolerance to enteral feeding is the rule. In some situations, parenteral nutrition via a peripheral vein may be effective, using a solution that does not exceed 900 mOsm/kg (e.g., 10% dextrose, 2% amino acids, and electrolytes). Peripheral solutions generally provide inadequate calories unless infused at a high rate. The administration of hyperosmolar solutions requires central venous access. The optimal location of the tip of the central venous catheter is at the junction of the superior vena cava and the right atrium.

- Initial infusion rates of these macronutrients generally begin at 2–4 mg/kg/min of carbohydrates, 0.5–1.0 g of amino acids/kg/day, and 1 g of lipids/kg/day.
- Electrolytes, minerals, trace elements, and a multivitamin preparation are generally added to the parenteral solution.
- With patients who are severely malnourished, overfeeding (by either enteral or parenteral route) may result in a refeeding syndrome characterized by electrolyte abnormalities (hypophosphatemia, hypokalemia, and hypomagnesemia), volume overload, and congestive heart failure. Refeeding syndrome is less likely if total parenteral nutrition is introduced gradually.

Complications of Total Parenteral Nutrition

- Mechanical complications may occur during central line placement. These include pneumothorax, brachial plexus injury, subclavian/carotid artery puncture, hemothorax, and chylothorax.

- Metabolic complications include fluid overload, hypertriglyceridemia, hypercalcemia, hypoglycemia, hyperglycemia, and specific nutrient deficiencies.
- Thrombosis or pulmonary embolism may occur. Radiologically evident subclavian vein thrombosis occurs commonly (25–50%), but clinically significant manifestations (e.g., upper extremity edema, superior vena cava syndrome, or pulmonary embolus) are rare. Inline filters should be used with all parenteral nutrient solutions.
- Infectious complications are most commonly caused by *Staphylococcus epidermidis* and *Staphylococcus aureus*.
- Hepatobiliary complications include elevated serum transaminases and alkaline phosphatase. In addition, steatosis, steatohepatitis, lipidosis and phospholipidosis, cholestasis, fibrosis, and cirrhosis may occur. Although these abnormalities are usually benign and transient, more serious and progressive disease may develop in a small subset of patients, usually after 16 wks of central parenteral nutrition.
- Metabolic bone disease may be seen with long-term total parenteral nutrition (>3 mos), including osteomalacia or osteopenia.

KEY POINTS TO REMEMBER

- There is no gold standard for evaluating the nutritional status of hospitalized patients. The best overall approach involves a thorough clinical and physical exam, a nutritional history, and appropriate lab studies.
- BMI is a useful indicator of nutritional status.
- Individuals who are severely malnourished at the outset of an illness often need nutritional support immediately, whereas patients with adequate stores can tolerate longer periods without adequate nutritional intake.
- If the gut works, use it.
- Parenteral nutrition should be given if the GI tract is not accessible or functional, as occurs in patients with bowel obstruction, ileus, necrotizing or inflammatory enterocolitis, severe pancreatitis, diffuse peritonitis, intractable vomiting, or short gut syndrome.

REFERENCES AND SUGGESTED READINGS

Kirby DF, Delegge MH, Fleming CR. AGA technical review on tube feeding for enteral nutrition. *Gastroenterology* 1995;108:1282–1301.

Koretz RL, Lipman TO, Klein S. AGA technical review on parenteral nutrition. *Gastroenterology* 2001;121:970–1001.

MacFie J. Enteral versus parenteral nutrition. *Br J Surg* 2000;87(9):1121–1122.

Muskat PC. The benefits of early enteral nutrition. In: Shikora SA, Blackburn GL, eds. *Nutrition support: theory and therapeutics*. New York: Chapman & Hall, 1997:231–241.

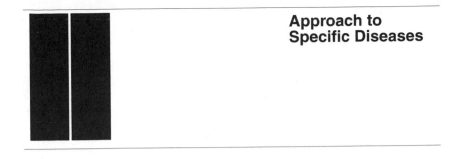

Approach to
Specific Diseases

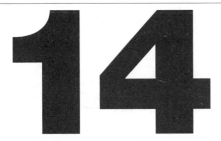

Esophageal Disorders

Dustin G. James

GASTROESOPHAGEAL REFLUX DISEASE

Gastroesophageal reflux disease (GERD) is extremely common and, if left untreated, can result in serious complications, such as esophageal stricture, hemorrhage, Barrett's esophagus, and adenocarcinoma. However, with the advent of *proton pump inhibitors (PPIs)*, most cases of GERD can be treated medically.

Causes

Pathophysiology

Reflux of acidic gastric contents into the esophagus is a normal event that occurs in healthy people. Prolonged exposure of the esophagus to gastric acid, however, is abnormal and often produces symptoms of GERD. There are several mechanisms that underlie reflux, almost all of which result in the failure of the gastroesophageal junction to prevent gastric contents from entering the esophagus. The gastroesophageal junction is composed of the lower esophageal sphincter (LES), the crural diaphragm, and the phrenoesophageal ligament. Most cases of GERD are related to either hypotensive or transient LES relaxations. Certain medications or endogenous chemicals may also decrease LES tone. In addition, impaired peristalsis allows refluxed contents to remain in contact with the esophageal mucosa. *Helicobacter pylori* infection does not contribute to reflux disease and may actually be protective. Regardless of the mechanism, the acid and enzymes present in gastric contents directly injure the squamous lining of the esophagus. Significant damage occurs when the esophagus is exposed to a pH of <4 for a prolonged period of time. Recent research suggests that reflux of duodenal contents, most notably bile, may also play an important role.

Presentation

The evaluation of GERD has three important aspects:

1. Cardiac diseases should be excluded, especially when chest pain is a symptom.
2. Workup should evaluate "alarm symptoms."
3. Severity of GERD should be assessed.

History and Physical Exam

The duration, frequency, and severity of heartburn should be determined. Because many patients with ischemic heart disease describe symptoms that are similar to GERD, the relationship of symptoms to exercise should be ascertained. Patients with GERD commonly report "acidic" taste in mouth and nocturnal wheezing or coughing. Other symptoms that may suggest GERD include hoarseness, chronic sore throat, or apnea. Behaviors that increase reflux should be sought, including smoking, caffeine use, large meals, and recumbency after eating. The presence of "alarm symptoms" should be determined, including dysphagia, weight loss, occult or overt GI bleeding, symptoms >5 yrs, age >45 yrs, and symptoms unresponsive to PPIs. The physical exam should assess body habitus (obesity) and check stool for occult blood.

Management

Lab Evaluation

Lab information is of limited use in the evaluation of GERD. A CBC may reveal a microcytic anemia if bleeding from esophagitis, cancer, or an erosion occurs.

Diagnostic Procedures

Although the degree of esophageal irritation does not always correlate with patient symptoms, many clinicians advocate a trial of a PPI to confirm the diagnosis in patients with suspected GERD. In the presence of "alarm symptoms," uncertainty of diagnosis, or inadequate response to PPI, further workup is necessary. Also, patients with long-standing GERD (>5–10 yrs) should have endoscopy performed to evaluate for Barrett's esophagus. Further workup often involves endoscopy, barium swallow, and 24-hr esophageal pH monitoring.

- Endoscopy may reveal esophagitis on gross exam, although many patients only have evidence of GERD on histologic exam. The main utility of esophagogastroduodenoscopy (EGD) is to evaluate for complications of GERD, such as stricture, hemorrhage, Barrett's esophagus, and adenocarcinoma.
- Barium swallow is often a low-yield exam, although reflux of barium from the stomach to the esophagus supports the diagnosis, and complications of GERD, such as strictures or masses, can be detected.
- Esophageal pH studies involve placement of an esophageal luminal pH monitor with measurement over a 24-hr period. This study is most useful in two clinical scenarios. If the diagnosis of GERD is in doubt, then monitoring can be performed off acid suppression. Generally, if the pH is <4 for ≥ 5% of the time, then the patient has GERD. Another use is in determining whether chest pain or other atypical symptoms are due to GERD. The pH study is performed to determine the adequacy of acid suppression in a patient with known GERD. This is performed with the patient on acid suppression. The patient is asked to record episodes of chest pain in a log. The correlation between chest pain and esophageal pH can then be determined.

Treatment

First-line therapy for moderate to severe GERD includes lifestyle modification and a PPI. The goal of treatment is to alleviate symptoms, heal the esophageal damage, and prevent the occurrence of complications of GERD.

- **Lifestyle modifications** include weight loss, smoking cessation, avoiding meals within 3 hrs of bedtime, and elevating the head of the patient's bed. Encourage patients to decrease consumption of alcohol, caffeine, and aggravating foods, such as onions and tomatoes. Patients should also avoid use of medications that lower LES tone, such as calcium channel blockers, beta blockers, nitrates, and anticholinergic drugs.
- **PPIs** given once daily can heal erosive esophagitis and relieve heartburn. In terms of efficacy, all of the PPIs are more effective than H_2-blockers or motility agents in healing esophageal lesions. If a once-daily dose is unsuccessful at relieving symptoms of GERD, or if patients have severe erosive esophagitis, strictures, ulcers, or Barrett's esophagus, the dose may be given twice daily with improved therapeutic benefit. If this dose does not relieve nocturnal symptoms, an H_2-blocker may be added at night to twice-daily PPI.
- **Surgical correction** is reserved for patients with documented GERD who do not respond to maximal medical therapy or do not wish to be on lifelong PPI.

Patients should undergo preoperative evaluation with motility studies and 24-hr pH monitoring. Recently, the surgical procedure most often used is laparoscopic Nissen fundoplication. Surgery is as effective as properly dosed PPI with less incidence of pulmonary aspiration. It entails more morbidity and mortality, however.

ESOPHAGEAL MALIGNANCIES

Esophageal squamous cell carcinoma and esophageal adenocarcinoma represent the two most common malignancies of the esophagus. In the United States, squamous cell carcinoma is decreasing in incidence, but the risk remains elevated in African-American men. There has been a troubling rise in the incidence of adenocarcinoma over the past 20 yrs. These diseases have a strong male predilection and a high mortality rate. Most patients have regional and distant lymph node metastases at the time of diagnosis.

Causes

Pathophysiology

SQUAMOUS CELL CARCINOMA OF THE ESOPHAGUS. Squamous cell carcinoma of the esophagus is the most common esophageal tumor worldwide. It is a leading cause of death in Central and Southeast Asia. In the United States, it is still relatively common in African-American men. Risk factors include chronic tobacco and alcohol use, chronic ingestion of hot liquids, history of mediastinal or breast irradiation, HPV 16 or 18 infection, and achalasia. The heavy use of both alcohol and tobacco smoke is a synergistic risk factor, increasing the risk of developing squamous cell carcinoma 100-fold. Carcinoma is believed to develop from carcinogenic exposure in susceptible individuals. The most common locations of disease are the proximal and distal esophagus, and incidence increases with advancing age.

ADENOCARCINOMA OF THE ESOPHAGUS. Several risk factors have been identified for adenocarcinoma, including Barrett's esophagus; GERD; obesity; scleroderma; history of colon cancer; and medications, including chronic use of theophylline or beta-agonists. Infection with *H. pylori* may have a protective effect. A large majority of cases occur near the gastroesophageal junction. Most cases present in obese middle-class men. It is believed that these risk factors cause the accumulation of genetic mutations in the normal squamous epithelium of the esophagus, leading to the development of adenocarcinoma.

BARRETT'S ESOPHAGUS. Barrett's esophagus represents the metaplasia of normal esophageal stratified squamous epithelium in the distal esophagus to specialized intestinal-type epithelium. Patients with Barrett's esophagus have a risk of developing esophageal adenocarcinoma that is approximately 100 times that of patients without the disease. Most cases of Barrett's esophagus occur in the setting of long-term, untreated GERD, occurring in approximately 10% of GERD patients. Bile reflux may also play an important role in the development of Barrett's esophagus. Most patients with GERD and Barrett's esophagus are symptomatic from GERD, but a significant population may be asymptomatic. Barrett's esophagus may progress from low-grade dysplasia to high-grade dysplasia and then adenocarcinoma, making treating of Barrett's and the underlying GERD very important.

Presentation

History and Physical Exam

A thorough history and physical exam should be performed. Key points to look for are a history of dysphagia and unintentional weight loss. Risk factors, especially country of origin, smoking history, and alcohol consumption, are useful in the diagnosis of squamous cell carcinoma. For adenocarcinoma, obesity and a history of GERD symptoms are useful. The stool should be tested for occult blood.

Management

Lab Evaluation
Lab tests provide little information to aid in the diagnosis of esophageal malignancies. Basic lab tests may reveal a microcytic anemia if bleeding has occurred. A low albumin may suggest malnutrition secondary to dysphagia.

Diagnostic Procedures
A barium swallow may reveal a mass in the esophageal lumen or compression from adjacent structures. EGD allows visualization of the esophageal lumen and biopsy of lesions and is the gold standard for diagnosis. Once the diagnosis of cancer has been established, the evaluation should focus on resectability, including endoscopic U/S and CT scan of the chest and abdomen to assess for local and distant spread. PET scanning is often useful to exclude distant metastases. However, many patients have local or distant spread at the time of diagnosis.

Treatment
SQUAMOUS CELL CARCINOMA. It is unclear if screening EGD is a cost-effective strategy in high-risk groups, such as those with a long history of alcohol and tobacco use or achalasia. The standard of care is surgery alone or in combination with radiation and chemotherapy. There is mounting evidence that adjuvant chemoradiotherapy plus surgery may be effective therapy. Patients often present with severe dysphagia that can be relieved with external-beam radiation therapy, surgical resection, or endoscopic stent placement.

ADENOCARCINOMA. The objective should be prevention or early detection of adenocarcinoma. The goal of PPI or surgical treatment should be not only relief of GERD symptoms, but also aggressive acid control. Despite acid control, few patients have complete regression of disease, making screening an important modality.

Once Barrett's esophagus is diagnosed, repeat endoscopic biopsies should be performed at 1- to 2-yr intervals. If low-grade dysplasia is found, follow-up is recommended in 6–12 mos. If high-grade dysplasia is found, the patient should be referred for possible esophagectomy. It is important to note that a large portion of patients referred to surgery with high-grade dysplasia may have undetected adenocarcinoma.

Surgical management of established cases of adenocarcinoma is similar to squamous cell carcinoma. Patients who are not surgical candidates should be offered palliative chemotherapy or radiation therapy. Survival rates for advanced esophageal cancer are extremely poor.

INFECTIOUS ESOPHAGITIS

With the advent of AIDS, the incidence of infectious esophagitis has increased, and the causal organisms have shifted over the past 20 yrs. The diagnosis of these diseases often requires endoscopic evaluation. However, many of these diseases have typical presentations and findings that may obviate invasive diagnosis.

Causes

Pathophysiology
IMMUNODEFICIENT HOST. Approximately 30% of patients with HIV infection have symptoms of esophageal infection during the course of their disease. These diseases become common as the T-cell CD4 count falls. However, almost all of these diseases are treatable; with highly active antiretroviral therapy, the incidence of these diseases is decreasing.

Fungal Esophagitis. Candidiasis is the most common infectious disease of the esophagus in HIV-infected patients, accounting for roughly 70% of all infections. The most common species is *Candida albicans*, but other species of *Candida* may be involved. Other fungi, such as *Histoplasma capsulatum*, can cause esophagitis, but these infections are rare. It is important to note that patients with AIDS may present with multiple esophageal infections at the same time. Almost all of these cases include *Candida* as one causal organism.

Viral Infection. The most common viral cause of esophagitis in HIV-infected patients is CMV. The risk of infection is low with CD4 counts >100 cells/μL. Unlike immunocompetent patients and those with immunodeficiency from other causes (e.g., organ transplant), herpes simplex virus (HSV) esophagitis is uncommon in HIV-infected patients. VZV can cause a devastating esophagitis in severely immunocompromised hosts. Other viruses, such as Epstein-Barr virus and papilloma, can infect the esophagus but are very rare.

Bacteria. Bacterial infection of the esophagus in HIV-infected patients is rare but can be seen. Pathogens involved are *Mycobacterium avium complex*, *Mycobacterium tuberculosis*, *Nocardia*, *Actinomyces*, and *Lactobacillus*.

Other. **Idiopathic esophageal ulceration (IEU)** is common in patients with a CD4 count <50 cells/μL. The etiologic agent of this disease has not been determined, although HIV itself has been implicated. In HIV-infected patients taking antiretroviral therapy, it is important to consider pill esophagitis as a cause of symptoms.

IMMUNOCOMPETENT HOST. HSV and VZV are the only common esophageal infections of the immunocompetent patient, although they are rare. HSV infection usually occurs in male patients and involves the mid-esophagus. VZV esophagitis often occurs in children with chickenpox or adults with herpes zoster.

Presentation

History and Physical Exam
A thorough history and physical exam should be performed, with emphasis on hydration status, nutritional status, and other key features listed below.

CANDIDIASIS. Dysphagia is the most common symptom of candidiasis. Odynophagia, fever, nausea, and vomiting are less common. Patients often have thrush. Up to one-half of patients with other esophageal infections and AIDS may have esophageal candidiasis as well.

CYTOMEGALOVIRUS. Odynophagia and esophagospasm are the most common symptoms of CMV. Patients may also have a low-grade fever and nausea and vomiting. Dysphagia is uncommon.

HERPES SIMPLEX VIRUS. Patients with HSV most commonly present with both odynophagia and dysphagia. Most infected patients also present with chest pain and fever.

VARICELLA ZOSTER VIRUS. The typical skin lesions of chickenpox in children or herpes zoster in adults may be seen. Otherwise, VZV presents similarly to HSV.

IDIOPATHIC ESOPHAGEAL ULCERATION. Almost all patients with IEU present with severe odynophagia and, as a result, are malnourished and dehydrated at presentation. The diagnosis is made when other etiologies have been ruled out.

Management

Lab Evaluation
An elevated WBC count on CBC may suggest infection, although this is variable in patients with immunodeficiency as compared to an immunocompetent host. The CD4 count is useful in determining which pathogen is likely involved in AIDS patients.

- >200: HSV, VZV
- 100–200: Candidiasis, HSV

- <100: Candidiasis, CMV, HSV
- <50: IEU

Diagnostic Procedures

Many clinicians recommend giving a patient with AIDS and dysphagia without other symptoms an empiric course of fluconazole, as *Candida* is the most likely pathogen. If the patient does not improve in 7 days or has other symptoms (e.g., weight loss, dehydration, or fever), further evaluation is needed. EGD is able to distinguish between the types of esophageal infections by gross or histologic appearance of the lesions.

CANDIDIASIS. Multiple adherent, white or yellow, "cottage cheese" plaques are easily seen on endoscopy. Brushings or biopsies reveal yeast or budding hyphae. Culture is useful in patients with a history of esophageal candidiasis for determining species and susceptibilities.

CYTOMEGALOVIRUS. Few large, well-demarcated ulcers are seen. Immunohistochemistry (special CMV staining) of biopsy aids in the diagnosis.

VARICELLA ZOSTER VIRUS. Multiple vesicles and confluent ulcers are seen. The cytology is difficult to distinguish from HSV and often requires immunohistochemistry or culture.

HERPES SIMPLEX VIRUS. HSV appears as either small, superficial ulcers or a diffuse esophagitis in later stages. Cytology reveals giant cells and ground-glass nuclei. Immunohistochemistry or culture confirms the diagnosis.

IDIOPATHIC ESOPHAGEAL ULCERATION. A few well-circumscribed, often large, ulcers are seen. Multiple biopsies should be taken to exclude other processes.

Treatment

CANDIDIASIS. First-line treatment is fluconazole, 200-mg oral loading dose, followed by 100 mg/day for a total of 5–10 days. Improvement is usually seen within a few days. In patients with azole-resistant *Candida*, the dose may be increased, or treatment with IV amphotericin can be initiated. Severe, refractory cases may not improve until treatment of HIV is undertaken to raise the CD4 count.

CYTOMEGALOVIRUS. First-line therapy includes IV ganciclovir, 5 mg/kg q12h, if the patient is not pancytopenic. Alternate therapy includes IV foscarnet, 60 mg/kg q8h. Treatment continues until healing occurs, usually up to 1 mo. Approximately 30% of patients relapse.

HERPES SIMPLEX VIRUS. First-line therapy includes IV acyclovir, 250 mg/m^2 q8h, then 200–400 mg, five doses/day for a total of 2 wks. Other effective agents are famciclovir, valacyclovir, and ganciclovir. Foscarnet is reserved for resistant strains because of its adverse effects.

VARICELLA ZOSTER VIRUS. High doses of IV acyclovir may be needed in refractory cases of VZV. Most, however, resolve spontaneously.

IDIOPATHIC ESOPHAGEAL ULCERATION. Treatment involves corticosteroids. Oral prednisone can be used; if the patient can not tolerate PO intake, then IV formulations are used. The use of corticosteroids often predisposes to *Candida* infection, and many clinicians also give fluconazole twice weekly as long as prednisone is given. Thalidomide is effective in treating IEU as well.

PROPHYLAXIS. Many of these diseases have high recurrence rates and warrant prophylaxis. Primary prophylaxis of *Candida* is not recommended; however, secondary prophylaxis in patients with multiple recurrences is used. Often, once weekly fluconazole, 100 mg PO, is effective. Although primary prevention of CMV is recommended in patients with CD4 counts <100, there are no data that support a decreased incidence of GI disease. Primary prophylaxis for HSV is not recommended. Secondary prophylaxis is recommended for patients with recurrent disease with acyclovir, 600 mg PO qd.

ESOPHAGEAL STRICTURES

Esophageal strictures often arise as complications of other disease processes. Any type of chronic inflammation can lead to esophageal strictures. Common causes include GERD, repetitive vomiting, caustic ingestion, infections, and pill esophagitis. Other, less common causes include NG tube injury, iron deficiency anemia, and Crohn's disease.

Causes

Pathophysiology

Strictures are the result of severe inflammation of the esophagus with resulting fibrosis or other reactive changes. Patients do not often develop symptoms of dysphagia until a significant amount of the esophageal lumen is obliterated. Peptic strictures are relatively common, occurring in approximately 10% of patients with GERD. Peptic strictures typically occur in the distal esophagus. Strictures as a result of esophageal infections, caustic ingestion, NG tube trauma, repetitive vomiting, or Crohn's disease often are more extensive. Lower esophageal (Schatzki's) rings often occur in the distal esophagus and are associated with GERD, pill esophagitis, and hiatal hernias. They are an extremely common cause of intermittent, solid food dysphagia. Plummer-Vinson syndrome includes iron deficiency, dysphagia, and upper esophageal webs and usually occurs in middle-aged women.

Presentation

History and Physical Exam

A careful history is crucial in the assessment of dysphagia. In addition to helping rule out diseases other than stricture, the type of dysphagia and regurgitation can often localize the site and involvement of disease. Key points of the history should include onset and duration of symptoms, association of dysphagia with type of foods, description of regurgitated material if present, history of weight loss, and history of GERD. Physical signs of weight loss, dehydration, and malnutrition help to assess severity. See Chap. 2, Dysphagia, for a discussion of the evaluation of suspected dysphagia.

Management

Lab Evaluation

Lab studies are not very useful in the workup of stricture. Iron-deficiency anemia may support the diagnosis of Plummer-Vinson syndrome. A low albumin may reflect nutritional deficiency.

Diagnostic Procedures

Barium swallow is a useful step in the workup of suspected stricture, ring, or web. Radiologic findings inconsistent with the patient's history warrant further evaluation with direct visualization with EGD. EGD is also useful for relieving identified areas of dysphagia with bougie or balloon dilation.

Treatment

SCHATZKI'S RING. Patients describe intermittent dysphagia for solids, often when eating meats or bread or when eating too quickly. In mild disease, patients should be advised to carefully masticate their food. Patients with more severe disease are at increased risk for food bolus impaction and benefit from passage of an endoscopic dilator. Refractory cases may require pneumatic dilation, electrocautery incision, or surgical repair. Patients should be assessed for GERD and treated with a PPI as needed.

PLUMMER-VINSON SYNDROME (ESOPHAGEAL WEB). Dysphagia is very responsive to iron repletion. Severe cases may require endoscopic dilation with bougienage. These patients have an increased risk of developing squamous cell carcinoma of the esophagus. It is unclear whether they should receive screening EGD.

PEPTIC STRICTURE. Aggressive acid control with high-dose PPI can cause regression of the stricture. Dilation of stricture, however, is often required. The dilation is performed endoscopically and may involve stents in severe cases. Occasionally, dysphagia is not relieved by maximum medical therapy, and surgery is required.

ESOPHAGEAL MOTILITY DISORDERS

Motility disorders of the esophagus can involve both the striated and smooth muscle of the esophagus. Often, dysfunction of one or multiple components of the esophageal neuromuscular system can be identified. These diseases can result in extreme morbidity for patients. Fortunately, new treatments are becoming available.

Causes

Pathophysiology

Swallowing involves two types of muscular activity. It is initiated by neural impulses from the CNS-controlling voluntary muscles of the oropharynx. It is completed by the involuntary contraction of the smooth muscle of the esophagus in a coordinated sequence. Dysfunction at any step can cause dysphagia.

STRIATED MUSCLE. The striated muscles of the oropharynx may be affected by a number of conditions, including cerebrovascular accidents, myasthenia gravis, polymyositis, Parkinson's disease, and amyotrophic lateral sclerosis. Neuromuscular dysregulation results in the loss of a coordinated swallow and can lead to dysphagia, regurgitation, and pulmonary aspiration. An inappropriately contracted cricopharyngeus muscle can lead to dysphagia in some patients.

SMOOTH MUSCLE

* The most common disease of smooth muscle function is **achalasia.** Achalasia results from the loss of inhibitory neurons in the esophagus. The loss leads to dysregulation of peristalsis and an increased LES tone. It can be primary or secondary due to invasive cancer or by infection by *Trypanosoma cruzi* causing Chagas' disease.
* Diffuse esophageal spasm (DES) and nutcracker esophagus are similar disorders of abnormal inhibitory neuron function that are nonprogressive.
* Scleroderma causes the smooth muscles of the distal esophagus to atrophy and LES tone to decrease. In early stages, it causes solid food dysphagia but can progress to severe dysphagia when complications of severe GERD develop.

Presentation

History and Physical Exam

The most common symptoms at presentation are dysphagia and chest pain. The history should focus on conditions that can cause motility disorders, such as cerebrovascular accident, amyotrophic lateral sclerosis, and myasthenia gravis. A history of travel to Central and South American countries may warrant workup for Chagas' disease. As with strictures, the type, duration, and severity of dysphagia are important to address. A description of regurgitated contents is useful as well. Complications of motility disorders, such as severe weight loss and aspiration pneumonia, should be assessed. Physical exam should include a thorough neurologic exam as well as assessment of nutritional status.

OROPHARYNGEAL DYSPHAGIA. Patients with oropharyngeal dysphagia often present with drooling, regurgitation of food immediately after swallowing, and pulmonary aspiration.

ACHALASIA. Achalasia often presents as progressive dysphagia and chest pain. Severe disease can result in solid and liquid dysphagia with accompanying weight loss. Patients often report a history of regurgitated, undigested food, often while sleeping.

NUTCRACKER ESOPHAGUS AND DIFFUSE ESOPHAGEAL SPASM. Patients present with nonprogressive, intermittent chest pain and dysphagia. It can range in severity from mild to extremely severe, sometimes with radiation to other parts of the body. Hence, it is important to rule out myocardial ischemia/infarct in patients with this presentation. Patients often have solid and liquid dysphagia, especially with very hot or cold items.

Management

Diagnostic Procedures

Radiologic and manometric data are very useful in diagnosing esophageal motility disorders.

ACHALASIA

• Barium swallow often reveals a characteristic "bird's beak" tapered distal esophagus with proximal dilation. This appearance can also occur with neoplastic compression of the lower esophagus (pseudoachalasia).

• Manometry reveals a lack of primary peristalsis and increased LES tone. If patients have simultaneous and repetitive contractions, the disease is termed *vigorous achalasia*.

• EGD should always be performed to exclude mass lesions as a cause of secondary achalasia or pseudoachalasia.

DIFFUSE ESOPHAGEAL SPASM

• Barium swallow often reveals a typical "corkscrew" or "rosary-bead" appearance. Nutcracker esophagus often appears normal.

• Manometry in DES reveals simultaneous contractions of the entire esophageal body. Nutcracker esophagus is defined by an elevated distal esophageal peristaltic amplitude.

• EGD often appears normal, although patients often have evidence of GERD.

Treatment

ACHALASIA. The only effective medical therapy is endoscopic botulinum toxin injection of the LES. Effectiveness requires repeated injections and can entail development of resistance and scarring. The standard nonsurgical treatment is with endoscopic esophageal dilation. Most patients experience immediate relief. There is a risk of esophageal perforation, however. Laparoscopy with surgical myotomy of the LES is gaining popularity; it has more long-term efficacy than other modalities of treatment. Patients with achalasia have an increased risk of squamous cell esophageal carcinoma (develops in 2–7%), and there is debate about whether regular surveillance EGD should be performed.

DIFFUSE ESOPHAGEAL SPASM. Patients with DES and GERD require reassurance that their disease is nonprogressive and not fatal. Psychiatric disorders are often comorbid with DES and nutcracker esophagus and should be considered. Medications such as nitrates and calcium channel blockers are often used in treatment. PPIs should also be included in the treatment regimen, given the strong link of GERD and these disorders. The use of dilation or pneumatic dilation is of limited value considering the episodic nature of these diseases. Laparoscopic surgical esophageal myotomy is indicated only in those patients with severe and refractory symptoms.

SCLERODERMA. Treatment of scleroderma should involve aggressive acid control with high-dose PPIs. The motor dysfunction is very refractory to treatment, however.

KEY POINTS TO REMEMBER

• During the evaluation of GERD, it is important to exclude other causes of chest pain—most important, cardiac causes.

• A trial of normal-dose, once-daily PPI is often used to confirm the diagnosis of uncomplicated GERD.

- Presence of dysphagia, weight loss, anemia, occult blood in stools, lack of response to PPI, or age >50 yrs warrants further evaluation with EGD.
- Once-daily PPI is the first-line treatment for GERD. It can be given twice daily if needed or an evening dose of H_2-blocker can be added to control nocturnal symptoms.
- In the United States, the incidence of esophageal adenocarcinoma is rising at an alarming rate.
- Patients with squamous cell carcinoma often have a long history of tobacco and alcohol use.
- Patients with adenocarcinoma are often obese and have a long history of GERD.
- Patients with Barrett's esophagus represent a high-risk group for development of esophageal adenocarcinoma and should be treated with aggressive acid control and endoscopic surveillance.
- Most cases of esophageal malignancy are advanced at the time of diagnosis and are thus associated with a high mortality rate.
- The most common causes of esophagitis in patients with AIDS are *Candida*, CMV, HSV, and IEU.
- Infections in an immunocompetent host are rare but can include HSV and VZV.
- Patients with suspected esophagitis who do not respond to an empiric trial of fluconazole or those with symptoms such as severe odynophagia or fever should undergo upper endoscopy.
- Peptic strictures are one of the most common complications of poorly controlled GERD.
- Schatzki's rings are the most common cause of intermittent solid food dysphagia.
- Striated muscle dysfunction often presents with difficulty swallowing in the context of known neuromuscular diseases. Treatment of underlying diseases and swallowing therapy are the most effective treatments.
- Achalasia typically presents as progressive dysphagia and chest pain. It can be treated with botulinum toxin injections, dilations, or surgery.
- Scleroderma should be managed with aggressive acid control to prevent serious sequelae of GERD.

REFERENCES AND SUGGESTED READINGS

Adler DG, Romero Y. Primary esophageal motility disorders. *Mayo Clin Proc* 2001;76 (2):195–200.

Bonacini M, Young T, Laine L. The causes of esophageal symptoms in human immunodeficiency virus infection: a prospective study of 110 patients. *Arch Intern Med* 1991;151:1567–1572.

DiPalma JA. Management of severe gastroesophageal reflux disease. *J Clin Gastroenterol* 2001;32(1):19–26.

Falk GW. Gastroesophageal reflux disease and Barrett's esophagus. *Endoscopy* 2001; 33(2):109–118.

Goyal RK. Diseases of the esophagus. In: Fauci AS, Braunwald E, Isselbacher KJ, et al., eds. *Harrison's principles of internal medicine*. New York: McGraw-Hill, 1998:1588–1596.

Heath EI, Forastiere AA, Limburg PJ, et al. Adenocarcinoma of the esophagus: risk factors and prevention. *Oncology* 2000;14(4):507–514.

Hetzel DJ, Dent J, Reed WD, et al. Healing and relapse of severe peptic esophagitis after treatment with omeprazole. *Gastroenterology* 1988;95:903–912.

Hoffman RM, Jaffee PE. Plummer-Vinson syndrome. *Arch Intern Med* 1995;155:2008–2011.

Klinkenberg-Know EC, Nelis F, Dent J, et al. Long-term omeprazole treatment in resistant gastroesophageal reflux disease: efficacy, safety, and influence on gastric mucosa. *Gastroenterology* 2000;118:661–669.

Lundell L, Miettinen P, Myrvold HE, et al. Continued follow-up of a randomized clinical study comparing antireflux surgery and omeprazole in gastroesophageal reflux disease. *J Am Coll Surg* 2001;192:172–181.

Streitz JM, Ellis FH, Gibb SP, et al. Achalasia and squamous cell carcinoma of the esophagus: analysis of 241 patients. *Ann Thorac Surg* 1995;59:1604–1609.

Wilcox CM, Monkemuller KE. Diagnosis and management of esophageal disease in the acquired immunodeficiency syndrome. *South Med J* 1998;91(11):1002–1007.

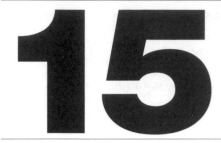

Gastric Disorders

Linda A. Cheng

PEPTIC ULCER DISEASE

Background

Gastric disorders, in particular peptic ulcer disease (PUD), are among the most common problems encountered by internists and gastroenterologists. PUD accounts for a significant portion of health care expenditures and imposes significant morbidity on many individuals.

Definition

PUD is characterized by denudation of mucosa exposed to gastric acid. By definition, this denudation extends into the muscularis propria layer. PUD most commonly occurs in the gastric antrum or duodenal bulb. Duodenal ulcers are more common than gastric ulcers.

Epidemiology

PUD is a worldwide problem. The lifetime risk of acquiring the disease is approximately 1 in 10. Duodenal ulcers are slightly more common in men than in women, but gastric ulcers occur with equal frequency among men and women. In the United States, there are approximately 500,000 new cases and 4 million recurrent cases of PUD each year. The annual mortality rate of PUD is low and is mostly due to complications, which include hemorrhage, perforation, and obstruction. Duodenal ulcer presents at a slightly younger age range than gastric ulcer: ages 25–55 yrs and ages 40–70 yrs, respectively. This difference is believed to be due to increased use of NSAIDs, which are associated primarily with gastric ulcers, in the elderly population.

Causes

Natural History

The natural history of PUD varies from resolution without treatment to recurrence with or without complications. Before the discovery in the 1980s of *Helicobacter pylori* infection as the most common cause of PUD, this disease was believed to be caused by stress, dietary factors, or gastric acid but frequently recurred despite treatment with antacids and antisecretory medications. Surgery was often performed for recurrent disease. Now, *H. pylori*–associated PUD is treated with eradication of *H. pylori*. As a result, the recurrence rate of PUD has markedly decreased, and elective surgery for PUD is exceedingly rare.

Differential Diagnosis

Etiologies for PUD are listed in Table 15-1. The most common forms of PUD are associated with *H. pylori* or the use of NSAIDs; these comprise 90% of cases of PUD. In patients in whom *H. pylori* infection, NSAID use, Crohn's disease, and Zollinger-Ellison syndrome have been ruled out, no apparent etiology is found in 50% of cases.

TABLE 15-1. FORMS OF PEPTIC ULCER DISEASE

Most common

   Helicobacter pylori–associated

   NSAID–associated

Other forms

   Stress ulcers

   Zollinger-Ellison syndrome

   Gastroduodenal Crohn's disease

   Viral infection

   Chemotherapy

   Radiation therapy

   Vascular insufficiency

Pathophysiology

The development of PUD is not entirely understood. It is believed to result from an imbalance of factors protective of the gastric mucosa, provided in part by prostaglandins and the mucous layer, and harmful factors, such as *H. pylori*, pepsin, NSAIDs, bile salts, and acid. Gastric ulcers are associated with normal or reduced levels of acid secretion, whereas duodenal ulcers are generally characterized by increased levels of acid secretion. Other factors that may play a role in PUD are elevated serum gastrin levels, increased acid output, and rapid gastric emptying, all of which have been associated with idiopathic PUD. A list of risk factors associated with PUD is found in Table 15-2.

***HELICOBACTER PYLORI*–ASSOCIATED PEPTIC ULCER DISEASE.** *H. pylori* infection has been associated with >90% of duodenal ulcers and 70–90% of gastric ulcers. It is also a risk factor for gastric adenocarcinoma and gastric mucosa–associated lymphoid tissue (MALT) lymphomas. The incidence of *H. pylori* in PUD appears to be decreasing, as more recent studies in the United States have demonstrated that 20–58% of ulcers are not associated with *H. pylori*. *H. pylori* infection is associated with lower socioeconomic status and is typically acquired in childhood.

    H. pylori is a gram-negative bacillus that lives in the mucous layer overlying gastric epithelium, leading to inflammation. It can also be found within epithelial cells and attached to mucous cells. In the case of duodenal ulcers, *H. pylori* is believed to infect ectopic gastric epithelium. The bacterium causes a diffuse gastritis and can be detected histologically in >90% of biopsies showing histologic inflammation in the stomach. This gastritis can cause hypochlorhydria or achlorhydria that may lead to PUD. In the case of gastric ulcers, *H. pylori* generally causes a severe pangastritis that leads to ulceration despite reduced acid secretion. With duodenal ulcers, the corpus of the stomach is relatively spared of inflammation, parietal cell function is intact, and ulceration occurs in the area of greatest inflammation.

    The ability of *H. pylori* to induce gastritis likely stems from a combination of qualities. The bacterium does not appear to have a predominant virulence factor.

TABLE 15-2. RISK FACTORS FOR PEPTIC ULCER DISEASE

Infection with *Helicobacter pylori*	Having a first-degree relative with peptic ulcer disease
Use of NSAIDs	
Smoking	Emigration from a developing nation
African-American or Hispanic ethnicity	

The bacterium secretes a **urease enzyme** that breaks down urea in the stomach to produce ammonia, which helps to neutralize the acidic gastric environment and thereby protect the organism. This urease activity provides the basis for many of the lab tests used to evaluate for *H. pylori* infection. In addition, *H. pylori* infection is believed to increase the permeability of the gastric mucous layer to pepsin and acid. Finally, the bacterium produces cytotoxins (CagA) that may also contribute to its pathogenicity.

NSAID-ASSOCIATED PEPTIC ULCER DISEASE. The second most common cause of PUD after *H. pylori* is NSAID use. NSAID use has been associated with 30–75% of *H. pylori*–negative ulcers and 15% of *H. pylori*–positive ulcers. The rate of GI complications in patients taking long-term NSAIDs varies from 7.3/1000 patients/yr for osteoarthritis to 13/1000 patients/yr for rheumatoid arthritis. NSAIDs have a direct toxic effect because of their acidic nature and because they can decrease the hydrophobicity of gastric mucus, allowing injury of the epithelium by acid and pepsin. However, the predominant mechanism for NSAID-associated PUD is inhibition of endogenous prostaglandin synthesis. As such, enteric-coated, parenteral, or rectal NSAIDs or ASA present the same risk of ulcers as their oral counterparts. Moreover, administration of NSAIDs with food does not decrease ulcer risk. Suppression of prostaglandin synthesis is mediated through inhibition of the cyclooxygenase (COX)-1 enzyme, which acts as a "housekeeping" enzyme to maintain the integrity of the gastric mucosa, where it is constitutively expressed. Inhibition of prostaglandin synthesis decreases mucus production, bicarbonate secretion, mucosal perfusion, and epithelial proliferation. This impairs the integrity of the mucosa, allowing damage by harmful factors like NSAIDs, pepsin, bile salts, and acid. Because the antiinflammatory effects of NSAIDs are believed to be mediated through the COX-2 enzyme, which is not expressed in the gastric mucosa, COX-2–selective inhibitors may be less likely to cause GI complications.

Risk factors for the development of NSAID-associated PUD include concomitant corticosteroid use, anticoagulants, and older age (Table 15-3). Corticosteroids alone are not a risk factor. The role of *H. pylori* infection in NSAID-associated PUD is at present unclear, with different studies showing conflicting results. However, it is generally believed that *H. pylori* and NSAIDs do not act synergistically to induce PUD.

NSAID use can cause a spectrum of lesions that may affect any area of the stomach, although the gastric antrum is most frequently involved. The various types of lesions seen range from superficial lesions to ulcers that are complicated by hemorrhage or perforation. Superficial lesions include petechiae and erosions, and these are likely due to direct toxic effects of NSAIDs and may occur within hours of NSAID administration. These lesions are confined to the mucosa and, as such, do not cause complications. Ulcers extend to the submucosa and are larger than erosions. Ulcers are found 10–25% of the time on endoscopy of NSAID users.

NSAID-associated ulcers are often complicated by hemorrhage and perforation. In fact, ≥ 60% of complicated gastroduodenal ulcers are associated with the use of NSAIDs or ASA. These complications occur with similar frequency among duodenal and gastric ulcers. Hemorrhage is the most common complication. Platelet dysfunction may contribute to the tendency toward hemorrhage, especially in the case of ASA. Hemorrhage

---

TABLE 15-3. RISK FACTORS FOR NSAID-ASSOCIATED PEPTIC ULCER DISEASE

Concomitant corticosteroid use	Prior peptic ulcer disease (associated with *Helicobacter pylori* or NSAIDs)
Concomitant bisphosphonate use	
Concomitant anticoagulant use	Increasing NSAID dose or prolonged use
Older age	Poor overall health
Female gender	

may occur at any time during the course of NSAID treatment, and the risk of hemorrhage at any given time does not change over an extended period of NSAID use.

ZOLLINGER-ELLISON SYNDROME. Gastrinoma, or the Zollinger-Ellison syndrome, accounts for only 0.1% of all peptic ulcers. The ulcers are caused by gastrin-producing endocrine tumors of the pancreas or duodenum. The increased gastrin levels cause histamine release from enterochromaffin-like cells in the gastric mucosa. The histamine then binds to histamine receptors on parietal cells, causing hypersecretion of hydrochloric acid. Peptic ulcers develop as the normal defense mechanisms against acid are overwhelmed by the high gastric acid output. Ulcers typically form in the duodenal bulb but may also be seen in the distal duodenum and jejunum, and multiple ulcers are commonly seen. The diagnosis should be suspected in any patient with multiple ulcers in unusual locations or patients with family history suggestive of possible multiple endocrine neoplasia type I. An elevated gastrin level suggests the diagnosis, and measurement of elevated fasting gastric acid output helps confirm the diagnosis.

Presentation

History
History alone is unreliable in diagnosing PUD. Approximately 70% of patients who report dyspepsia have nonulcer dyspepsia, and up to 40% of patients with active PUD have no abdominal pain. However, the classic symptoms that would suggest PUD are episodes of burning or dull nonradiating epigastric pain that improve with antacids or food. Pain typically comes on with hunger or hours after eating. Pain may also occur at nighttime and is intermittent, recurring over months to years. The patient may experience associated nausea or vomiting.

Patients should be questioned carefully about NSAID and ASA use, including over-the-counter NSAIDs. Even if patients have discontinued NSAIDs, they may still present with GI toxicity up to 1 yr later. NSAID-associated ulcers are more likely than other forms of peptic ulcers to be painless and may present initially with bleeding rather than dyspepsia.

Physical Exam
In the absence of complicated PUD, physical exam is not very helpful. Patients may have epigastric tenderness. However, the sensitivity, specificity, positive predictive value, and negative predictive value of epigastric tenderness on deep palpation are ≤ 50%. Patients with perforated peptic ulcers usually exhibit signs of peritonitis. Patients with bleeding ulcers may have fecal occult blood, melena, or hematemesis. If they are hemodynamically compromised, they may be tachycardic or hypotensive.

Management

Diagnostic Evaluation
Routine lab studies are usually unremarkable. CBC may show iron-deficiency anemia from chronic fecal occult blood loss or anemia from acute blood loss.

Patients in whom PUD is suspected should be tested for *H. pylori* infection. Patients with a history of documented peptic ulcer or gastric MALT lymphoma should also be tested, although some would argue that the likelihood of *H. pylori* infection in individuals with no history of NSAID use and a history of documented PUD is so high that testing is unnecessary. As a corollary, patients should not be tested for *H. pylori* infection unless treatment is intended. Moreover, asymptomatic patients without a history of PUD and patients on long-term treatment with proton pump inhibitors (PPIs) for gastroesophageal reflux disease do not need to be tested.

Several types of tests have been developed to detect the presence of *H. pylori*. These tests include *serology*, *urease assays*, and *histology*. Some of these tests are noninvasive, whereas others require endoscopy. The decision regarding which test to perform and whether to perform endoscopy depends on the individual patient. Culture is not generally performed because it is expensive, time consuming, and difficult. Culture should not be considered unless a patient does not respond to eradication treatment and there is concern about antibiotic resistance.

SEROLOGY. Serology tests for IgG antibodies to *H. pylori*. Serology diagnoses *H. pylori* infection rather than the presence of PUD per se. Because of their high sensitivity, serologic tests perform best in areas with a high prevalence of *H. pylori*. The most common serologic tests are lab-based ELISA tests. Less commonly used serology tests are based on immunochromatography and Western blotting. The accuracy of ELISA testing can extend up to 95%. Serologic testing is inexpensive, but antibodies may remain positive for >1 yr after treatment of the infection, so it is difficult to evaluate *H. pylori* infection with serology after treatment.

UREASE ASSAYS. Urease assays test for the presence of the urease enzyme, which is produced in high amounts by *H. pylori*. These tests include noninvasive urease breath testing and biopsy urease tests. They can be used both to diagnose active infection and to confirm cure of *H. pylori* infection. False-negative results may occur in the setting of treatment with PPIs, H_2-receptor blockers, antibiotics, or bismuth-containing medications. Therefore, PPIs should be held for 7–14 days before testing. In addition, urease breath testing to confirm cure of *H. pylori* should be held until 4 wks after completing treatment for *H. pylori* infection.

The urea breath test is the best noninvasive method of diagnosing *H. pylori* infection. There are two forms of urea breath tests: the ^{14}C-urea breath test and ^{13}C-urea breath test. The two breath tests use urea that has been labeled with either a radioactive (^{14}C) or nonradioactive (^{13}C) isotope. Labeled urea is given orally to the patient; in the presence of urease, the urea is broken down into ammonia and labeled CO_2. After absorption of CO_2 into the circulation, it is expelled into the breath. $^{13}CO_2$ is detected by mass spectroscopy, whereas $^{14}CO_2$ is detected by scintillation counting. Radioactive urea breath testing is contraindicated in pregnant women and in children. The theoretic advantage of urea breath testing over biopsy urease tests is a decreased number of false-negative tests due to sampling error.

Biopsy urease tests include the CLOtest, Pyloritek, and Hp-fast. Biopsy urease testing is the best endoscopic method of diagnosing *H. pylori*. Most of these tests involve a pH-sensitive dye that changes color due to an increase in pH secondary to the production of ammonia from urea. In addition to false-negative results in the setting of prior treatment with PPIs, false-negative results may occur if blood from recent or active bleeding is present. If it is not possible to hold PPIs before testing, biopsies should be taken from both the antrum and the fundus to increase the likelihood of a positive result.

HISTOLOGY. Histology is not usually necessary to diagnose *H. pylori* infection. Histology requires the performance of endoscopy. It is indicated in gastric ulcers due to the risk of malignancy or in cases of PUD in which urease testing might be falsely negative (e.g., in the setting of use of PPIs before endoscopy). In the case of gastric ulcers, biopsies should be obtained from around the ulcer crater to rule out malignancy, but they should be obtained from other areas of the stomach to test for *H. pylori*. Biopsy may be less sensitive in the setting of bleeding ulcers, so other sampling-independent testing, such as serology, should be performed. Patients with a gastric ulcer should undergo follow-up endoscopy at 8–12 wks to document ulcer healing and exclude malignancy. Duodenal ulcers do not require biopsy because of the extremely low risk of malignancy.

***HELICOBACTER PYLORI* TESTING IN COMPLICATED PEPTIC ULCER DISEASE.** *H. pylori* testing is more likely to be negative in complicated PUD. Among patients with bleeding duodenal ulcers, only 70% are infected with *H. pylori*. Moreover, in one study among patients with perforated peptic ulcers, only 50% were infected. The lower rate of *H. pylori* in complicated PUD may be at least partially due to a higher false-negative rate for biopsy urease tests. Therefore, a negative biopsy urease test in the case of a complicated peptic ulcer warrants additional testing for *H. pylori*. If the patient has never undergone treatment for *H. pylori*, serology is the test of choice in the setting of PUD complicated by hemorrhage.

ENDOSCOPY. Decisions regarding endoscopy in patients with symptoms of PUD should be made based on patients' symptoms and the risk of gastric cancer. If there is high suspicion of PUD based on history and exam, consideration may be given to performing noninvasive testing, such as serology and urease breath testing without endoscopy, especially if the patient is relatively young and otherwise healthy. These tests are more cost-effective than esophagogastroduodenoscopy. However, endoscopy should be performed in patients who have signs or symptoms worrisome for gastric cancer. These include anorexia, dysphagia, epigastric mass, severe vomiting, weight loss, anemia, advanced age, and family history of upper GI cancer. Patients with significant dyspepsia, acute GI bleeding, fecal occult blood, or abdominal pain of unclear etiology should also undergo endoscopy. Gastric ulcers should be biopsied to rule out gastric cancer.

Treatment

Medications used to treat PUD include antisecretory drugs and mucosal protectants such as sucralfate. Antisecretory drugs include histamine$_2$ (H$_2$)-receptor antagonists, PPIs, and prostaglandin analogues. H$_2$-receptor antagonists inhibit acid secretion by blocking the binding of histamine to its receptor on the parietal cell. They inhibit both basal and food-induced acid secretion. The H$_2$-receptor blockers available in the United States include cimetidine, famotidine, nizatidine, and ranitidine. This class of drugs is well tolerated, although doses should be adjusted in patients with renal insufficiency. In general, when used in the treatment of gastroduodenal ulcer disease, H$_2$-blockers are most effective when administered between dinner and bedtime. PPIs are prodrugs that, when activated by acid, bind to and inhibit the parietal cell H$^+$/K$^+$-ATPase. Because they require acid for activation, they are most effectively taken before or with a meal and in the absence of other antisecretory drugs. PPIs pose a theoretic risk of inducing enterochromaffin-like cell hyperplasia and carcinoid tumors, but these drugs have been used safely in the United States for the past decade without a notable increase in the incidence of carcinoid tumors. Misoprostol is a prostaglandin analog that inhibits acid secretion. It is the only drug that has been approved by the FDA for prophylaxis of NSAID-induced peptic ulcers. Due to its mechanism of action, misoprostol may cause diarrhea or spontaneous abortion.

HELICOBACTER PYLORI–ASSOCIATED PEPTIC ULCER DISEASE. Patients with documented *H. pylori* infection should be treated with antibiotics and antisecretory therapy. Treatment of *H. pylori* infection with antibiotics significantly lowers the recurrence rate. Patients treated with antisecretory therapy alone have a recurrence rate of 60–100%, compared to <15% in patients treated with *H. pylori* eradication.

A number of regimens have been developed for *H. pylori* eradication, mostly through trial and error. Because *H. pylori* is difficult to eradicate, effective *H. pylori* regimens usually involve more than one antibiotic and ≥ 10 days of therapy. Some regimens are relatively inexpensive but require qid dosing, which may decrease compliance. Because most regimens involve ≥ 2 antibiotics, they may also be associated with unpleasant side effects. Accepted treatment regimens are listed in Table 15-4.

Of note, amoxicillin and clarithromycin are pH-dependent antibiotics that work more effectively in combination with antisecretory drugs. These regimens include multiple antibiotics to maximize the likelihood of eradication and to prevent the spread of antimicrobial resistance. Monotherapy is inadequate. Even so, none of these regimens eradicates *H. pylori* in all patients. In general, the eradication rate is 70–90%. *H. pylori* therapy may be unsuccessful because of noncompliance or antibiotic resistance. In the United States, resistance most commonly occurs with metronidazole or clarithromycin.

In addition to antibiotics, patients should also be treated with antisecretory therapy. It is debated as to whether antisecretory medications accelerate the rate of healing. However, they do allow faster resolution of symptoms. The course of antisecretory treatment depends on the location of the ulcer. Duodenal ulcers should be treated for 4 wks, and gastric ulcers should be treated for 8 wks. In general, with ulcers >1 cm, it is reasonable to treat with a longer course of antisecretory therapy.

TABLE 15-4. TREATMENT REGIMENS FOR *HELICOBACTER PYLORI* ERADICATION

OAC	Omeprazole, 20 mg PO bid; amoxicillin, 1000 mg PO bid; clarithromycin, 500 mg PO bid
LAC	Lansoprazole, 30 mg PO bid; amoxicillin, 1000 mg PO bid; clarithromycin, 500 mg PO bid
HBMT	H_2-receptor blocker, PO bid; bismuth subsalicylate, 525 mg PO qid; metronidazole, 500 mg PO qid; tetracycline, 250 mg PO qid
RBC	Ranitidine bismuth citrate, 400 mg PO bid (28 d); clarithromycin, 500 mg PO bid (14 d)

Note: Treatment durations range from 10 to 14 days for OAC, LAC, and HBMT. As noted, ranitidine bismuth citrate should be given for 28 days. Eradication rates of 70–90% are seen with these FDA-approved regimens.

CONFIRMATION OF *HELICOBACTER PYLORI* ERADICATION. In patients with uncomplicated PUD, confirmation of cure is not required because recurrence would most likely also be uncomplicated. However, testing for *H. pylori* eradication should be performed in patients with recurrent symptoms, complicated PUD, gastric MALT lymphoma, or early gastric cancer. Because of the high rate of bleeding recurrence in untreated *H. pylori*–positive bleeding ulcers, testing for eradication is critical. Confirmation of cure can be performed by urea breath testing. In the case of *H. pylori*–positive complicated PUD, testing for cure of *H. pylori* should be done after treatment to minimize recurrence. To avoid false-negative results, urea breath testing should be performed ≥ 4 wks after the end of *H. pylori* therapy and 2 wks after finishing treatment with PPIs. Serology testing to document eradication is less useful, as the antibody may remain positive for up to 1 yr after successful eradication.

NSAID-ASSOCIATED PEPTIC ULCER DISEASE. For patients with NSAID-associated PUD, consideration should be given to stopping the offending drug, as continuation of NSAID use delays ulcer healing. However, discontinuing NSAIDs is not always practical. In patients who must continue to take NSAIDs, GI toxicity may be reduced by decreasing the dose or switching to a less gastrotoxic medication, such as a COX-2 inhibitor. Concomitant corticosteroid, anticoagulant, or bisphosphonate therapy should be discontinued if possible.

Direct treatment of NSAID-induced ulcers is acid suppression with an H_2-receptor antagonist or a PPI. Studies have shown that even with continued NSAID use, approximately 75% of gastric ulcers and 87% of duodenal ulcers heal after 6–12 wks of treatment with conventional doses of H_2-receptor antagonists. Continuation of NSAID use does result in delayed healing, and larger ulcers also take longer to heal. A number of trials comparing PPIs to H_2-receptor antagonists in patients with NSAID-induced ulcer disease who continue to take NSAIDs have demonstrated higher rates of ulcer healing with PPIs than H_2-receptor antagonists. Therefore, the current recommendation is to treat NSAID-associated ulcers with PPIs if the patient is to continue to take NSAIDs. PPI therapy should continue as long as the patient is being treated with NSAIDs to reduce the risk of ulcer recurrence.

RECURRENT PEPTIC ULCER DISEASE. The most important risk factors for ulcer recurrence are *H. pylori* infection and NSAID use. Among untreated bleeding *H. pylori*–positive peptic ulcers, approximately one-third present with recurrent bleeding within 1 yr. Likewise, treatment of *H. pylori* dramatically reduces the rate of recurrent disease. The incidence of *H. pylori* reinfection after eradication is very low in developed countries.

MAINTENANCE ANTISECRETORY THERAPY. Maintenance antisecretory therapy after treatment of *H. pylori* infection is not cost-effective and is generally unnecessary in the treatment of PUD. It may be considered in high-risk cases, such as patients with

TABLE 15-5.
RISK FACTORS FOR GASTRIC ADENOCARCINOMA

Helicobacter pylori infection	Prior gastrectomy
Chronic atrophic gastritis	Blood type A
Pernicious anemia	Family history of gastric cancer
Gastric adenoma	Low socioeconomic status

complicated PUD, patients with *H. pylori*–negative ulcer disease, and patients in whom *H. pylori* eradication is unsuccessful.

GASTRIC ADENOCARCINOMA

In the early 1900s, stomach cancer was the most common cancer in the United States. Over the last 80 years, the incidence has decreased dramatically for unclear reasons. However, gastric cancer remains a major cause of death in other parts of the world, necessitating routine screening in Japan, for example. Multiple risk factors for gastric cancer have been identified (Table 15-5).

Presentation

Many patients with gastric cancer are asymptomatic or have nonspecific symptoms, including indigestion, epigastric discomfort, anorexia, early satiety, and weight loss. By the time symptoms have been investigated, many gastric cancers are advanced. Physical exam may reveal an epigastric mass, ascites, occult blood in the stool, or lymphadenopathy. An enlarged left supraclavicular node (Virchow's node) or periumbilical lymph node (Sister Mary Joseph's node) represents a metastatic site.

Management

Diagnostic Evaluation
Lab evaluation is of limited use but may demonstrate iron-deficiency anemia from chronic blood loss from the cancer. Diagnosis is best made with upper endoscopy, as this allows direct visualization as well as tissue sampling. Most gastric cancers are exophytic or fungating masses, but some manifest as nonhealing ulcers or with perforation of the gastric wall. All gastric ulcers should be aggressively biopsied to exclude malignancy. Repeat esophagogastroduodenoscopy should be performed at 8–12 wks in any patient with a gastric ulcer to document healing. Once the diagnosis of gastric adenocarcinoma is established, staging should be performed with endoscopic U/S or abdominal CT scans to determine whether surgical resection is an option.

Treatment
Surgical resection offers the only chance for cure. However, most cancers are unresectable due to local or metastatic spread at the time of diagnosis. Depending on location, partial or total gastrectomy may be performed. Even with complete resection, 5-yr survival is only approximately 20%. Palliative chemotherapy can be given to patients who are not surgical candidates, but the median survival is only 6–9 mos.

KEY POINTS TO REMEMBER

- The most common forms of PUD are associated with *H. pylori* or the use of NSAIDs. These comprise 90% of cases of PUD.

- Gastric ulcers should be biopsied to rule out malignancy. Most patients should undergo repeat endoscopy at 8–12 wks to document ulcer healing.
- Treatment of *H. pylori* dramatically reduces recurrence of PUD.
- In patients with uncomplicated PUD, confirmation of cure is not required because recurrence would most likely also be uncomplicated. However, testing for *H. pylori* eradication should be performed in patients with recurrent symptoms, complicated PUD, gastric MALT lymphoma, or early gastric cancer.
- The current recommendation is to treat NSAID-associated ulcers with PPIs if the patient is to continue to take NSAIDs. PPI therapy should continue as long as the patient is being treated with NSAIDs to reduce the risk of ulcer recurrence.
- Many patients with gastric cancer are asymptomatic or have nonspecific symptoms, including indigestion, epigastric discomfort, anorexia, early satiety, and weight loss.
- Palliative chemotherapy can be given to patients with gastric cancer who are not surgical candidates, but the median survival is only 6–9 mos.

REFERENCES AND SUGGESTED READINGS

Cappell MS, Schein JR. Diagnosis and treatment of nonsteroidal anti-inflammatory drug-associated upper gastrointestinal toxicity. *Gastroenterol Clin North Am* 2000; 29:97–124.

Cohen H. Peptic ulcer and *Helicobacter pylori*. *Gastroenterol Clin North Am* 2000;29: 775–789.

Graham DY. Therapy of *Helicobacter pylori*: current status and issues. *Gastroenterology* 2000;118:S2–S8.

Howden CW, Hunt RH. Guidelines for the management of *Helicobacter pylori* infection. *Am J Gastroenterol* 1998;93:2330–2338.

McColl KEL. *Helicobacter pylori*-negative ulcer disease. *J Gastroenterol* 2000;35 [Suppl XII]:47–50.

Soll A, Isenberg J. Peptic ulcer disease: epidemiology, pathophysiology, clinical manifestations, and diagnosis. In: Goldman L, Bennett JC, eds. *Cecil textbook of medicine*, 21st ed. Philadelphia: WB Saunders, 2000;671–675.

Walsh JW, Peterson WL. The treatment of *Helicobacter pylori* infection in the management of peptic ulcer disease. *N Engl J Med* 1995;333:984–991.

Wolfe MM, Lichtenstein DR, Singh G. Gastrointestinal toxicity of nonsteroidal anti-inflammatory drugs. *N Engl J Med* 1999;340:1888–1899.

Wolfe MM, Sachs G. Acid suppression: optimizing therapy for gastroduodenal ulcer healing, gastroesophageal reflux disease, and stress-related erosive syndrome. *Gastroenterology* 2000;118:S9–S31.

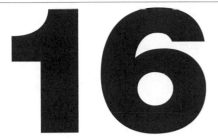

Small Bowel Disorders

Varsha V. Shah

INTRODUCTION

The small bowel is approximately 300–800 cm in length, but the functional surface area is >600 times that of a hollow tube. The villi, microvilli, and folds in the mucosa help contribute to this huge area for digestion, absorption, and secretion. Diseases of the small intestine generally result in problems with malabsorption and maldigestion. Consequently, the clinical manifestations of small bowel disorders reflect deficiencies of various macro- and micronutrients.

MALABSORPTION

Causes

Small bowel disorders, pancreatic exocrine insufficiency, and cholestatic liver disease account for most causes of malabsorption. Table 16-1 lists the most common etiologies of malabsorption. Pancreatic disease and liver disease are discussed individually in Chap. 20, Acute Liver Disease; Chap. 21, Chronic Liver Disease; Chap. 22, Cirrhosis; and Chap. 23, Pancreatic Disorders.

Presentation

Many patients with malabsorption present with weight loss despite a good appetite. In addition, most patients have an increased number of stools, which are foul-smelling with an oily character, making them difficult to flush. Malabsorption of specific fat-soluble vitamins leads to various clinical findings, including night blindness (vitamin A), osteopenia (vitamin D), or bleeding diathesis (vitamin K). Iron deficiency may develop, as the duodenum is the site for most iron absorption. Abdominal distention, flatulence, and abdominal cramps are common with carbohydrate malabsorption. Other common nonspecific findings include fatigue, muscle wasting, edema, amenorrhea, and orthostatic hypotension. Other, more specific clinical findings are discussed with the respective diseases below.

Management

There are a number of tests that may be useful in the evaluation of the patient with suspected small bowel disease.

Fecal Fat Analysis

The fecal fat analysis should be performed in all patients with suspected malabsorption. Qualitative analysis using Sudan staining is a good screening test but should be confirmed with quantitative analysis. This involves measurement of fat content for 24–72 hrs while the patient is on a 100-g fat diet. Normal fat absorption is >95% efficient, so <5 g/day indicates normal fat absorption. This test does not distinguish between small bowel disorders, pancreatic exocrine insufficiency, or cholestatic liver disorders.

TABLE 16-1. CAUSES OF MALABSORPTION

Small intestine disorders	Pancreatic exocrine insufficiency
Celiac sprue	Chronic pancreatitis
Tropical sprue	Cystic fibrosis
Short bowel syndrome	Pancreatic cancer
Radiation enteritis	Cholestatic liver disease
Small bowel lymphoma	Extrahepatic biliary obstruction
Amyloidosis	Intrahepatic biliary obstruction
Abetalipoproteinemia	Cirrhosis
Ileal resection	
Whipple disease	
AIDS	
Crohn's disease	
Diabetes mellitus	
Bacterial overgrowth	

Xylose Absorption Test

If a patient has an abnormal quantitative fat analysis, the xylose absorption test is useful to determine whether a small bowel disorder is present. Xylose is absorbed by passive diffusion across the small intestine, so abnormal xylose absorption indicates impaired intestinal absorption. The patient is given 25 g of xylose orally, and urinary excretion, hydrogen breath testing, or serum concentration of xylose is then measured.

Small Bowel Barium Studies

Generally, imaging studies are of limited use in suspected cases of small bowel disorders. However, specific findings may be helpful, including ileal strictures (Crohn's disease), mucosal thickening (lymphoma), fistulas, and diverticula (bacterial overgrowth).

Endoscopic Biopsy

Biopsy of the small intestine is extremely useful in patients with suspected malabsorption. Specific histologic findings allow diagnosis of many of the common causes of malabsorption, especially celiac sprue, lymphoma, and amyloidosis.

CELIAC SPRUE

Causes

Celiac sprue, also known as *celiac disease* or *gluten-sensitive enteropathy*, is a chronic malabsorptive disorder of the small intestine. It is characterized by villous atrophy and is caused by exposure to dietary gluten. It is relatively common in Western Europe, where up to 1 in 250 individuals has the disease. It is less common in the United States. It was previously believed to be a disorder of children, but adult presentation is common, and it can occur at any age. There is a strong association with certain HLA-DQ alleles. The exact mechanism for villous flattening is unknown, but it is believed that T cells are activated by specific components of gluten, resulting in damage to the small intestinal villi.

Presentation

Patients with celiac sprue may present with symptoms consistent with malabsorption, including weight loss, fatigue, abdominal cramps, and steatorrhea; however, anemia (iron, folate, or B_{12} deficiency), osteoporosis (calcium or vitamin D malabsorption), or infertility may be the only manifestation in adults. Other associated conditions include insulin-dependent diabetes mellitus, Sjögren syndrome, splenic atrophy, and thyroid disease. Dermatitis herpetiformis is an extraintestinal manifestation of gluten-sensitive enteropathy. This presents as a pruritic, blistering rash.

Management

Diagnostic Evaluation

Testing for patients with suspected celiac sprue should begin with scrum testing for tissue transglutaminase antibody. If positive, celiac sprue is very likely, and small bowel biopsy should be performed to document the presence of villous atrophy and lymphocytic infiltrate. If the tissue transglutaminase antibody is negative, celiac sprue is less likely, and other causes of malabsorption should be considered. In this case, small bowel biopsy often proves useful to exclude celiac sprue and look for other small bowel disorders.

Treatment

Treatment of celiac sprue involves strict adherence to a gluten-free diet. This often proves very difficult, as many different foods contain gluten. Patients should remove wheat, rye, and barley from the diet. Assistance from a dietitian is helpful to educate the patient on foods that should be avoided. The most common reason for resistant disease is noncompliance with a gluten-free diet. Monitoring of tissue transglutaminase antibody titers may help to verify dietary compliance. If symptoms persist despite complete removal of gluten, other diagnoses should be considered. There may be a role for steroids, 6-mercaptopurine, or azathioprine in refractory disease.

In addition to avoidance of gluten, specific nutrient deficiencies should be determined and corrected. There is an increase in overall mortality in patients with celiac sprue. This may be due to the slightly increased incidence of small bowel lymphoma. The risk of lymphoma normalizes after a 5-yr gluten-free period.

SHORT BOWEL SYNDROME

Resection of small intestine reduces the absorptive surface area. Depending on the length of bowel resected, this may cause no symptoms or may result in severe malabsorption. The length of remaining small intestine determines the severity of disease. Generally, patients with <100 cm suffer from malabsorption. In addition, surgeries that result in loss of the ileocecal valve cause more significant disease. Crohn's disease, mesenteric infarction, and trauma are the most common reasons for extensive small bowel resections. The diagnosis is usually relatively simple, as patients present with symptoms of malabsorption, volume depletion, or specific nutrient deficiencies in the setting of prior bowel resection. The specific nutrient deficiencies depend on the specific segment of bowel resected. Extensive jejunal resection results in folate, calcium, and iron malabsorption despite hyperplasia of the ileum. Ileal resection causes depletion of bile salts and vitamin B_{12} due to loss of specific receptors in the terminal ileum.

Treatment of small bowel syndrome depends on the length of remaining intestine and the specific segments that have been resected. Attempts should always be made to maintain nutrition via enteral intake. This involves supplementation with minerals and vitamins. To increase absorptive time, diphenoxylate-atropine or loperamide can be used to slow GI tract motility. In the event that adequate nutrition and fluid intake cannot be maintained with oral intake, long-term total parenteral nutrition may be required.

SMALL BOWEL TUMORS

Adenomas

Because of the risk of malignancy, all adenomas in the small intestine should be resected. The type of resection depends on the location of the tumor. Duodenal polyps can generally be resected endoscopically, and local resection is adequate. Periampullary tumors can also be removed endoscopically but often require surgical management due to the increased risk of malignancy.

Adenocarcinoma

Although the small intestine comprises 75% of the length of the entire GI tract and 90% of the mucosal surface, only 1% of adenocarcinomas of the GI tract arise from the small bowel. Adenocarcinoma is the most common small bowel malignancy, most commonly presenting in the sixth or seventh decade. The duodenum is the most common location for small bowel adenocarcinoma. Surgery provides the only potential for cure, and pancreaticoduodenectomy (Whipple procedure) is often required for tumors of the first or second part of the duodenum. Chemotherapy and radiation therapy have not been shown to improve survival in patients with advanced disease.

Lymphoma

Primary small bowel lymphomas account for 12–24% of small bowel malignancies. B-cell non-Hodgkin's lymphoma is the most common primary intestinal lymphoma. These patients often present with abdominal pain, weight loss, abdominal mass, perforation, or obstruction. The diagnosis can occasionally be made with small bowel biopsy, but exploratory laparotomy may be required to confirm the diagnosis. Most patients present with advanced disease and often require combined therapy with surgery, chemotherapy, or radiation therapy.

KEY POINTS TO REMEMBER

- Small bowel disorders, pancreatic exocrine insufficiency, and cholestatic liver disease account for most causes of malabsorption.
- Fecal fat analysis should be performed in all patients with suspected malabsorption.
- Treatment of celiac sprue involves strict adherence to a gluten-free diet.
- The length of remaining small intestine determines the severity of disease in short bowel syndrome. Generally, patients with <100 cm suffer from malabsorption.
- Ileal resection causes depletion of bile salts and vitamin B_{12} due to loss of specific receptors in the terminal ileum.
- Although the small intestine comprises 75% of the length of the entire GI tract and 90% of the mucosal surface, only 1% of adenocarcinomas of the GI tract arise from the small bowel.

REFERENCES AND SUGGESTED READINGS

Allard JP, Jeejeebhoy KN. Nutritional support and therapy in the short bowel syndrome. *Gastroenterol Clin North Am* 1980;18:589.

Buchman AL, Scolapio J, Fryer J. AGA technical review on short bowel syndrome and intestinal transplantation. *Gastroenterology* 2003;124:1111.

Ciclitira PJ. AGA technical review on celiac sprue. *Gastroenterology* 2001;120:1526.

Darling RC, Welch CE. Tumors of the small intestine. *N Engl J Med* 1959;260:397.

Lennard-Jones JE. Review article: practical management of the short bowel. *Aliment Pharmacol Ther* 1994;8:563.

Miles RM, Crawford D, Duras S. The small bowel tumor problem. *Ann Surg* 1979; 189:732.

Thompson JS. Management of the short bowel syndrome. *Gastroenterol Clin North Am* 1994;23:403.

Trier JS. Diagnosis of celiac sprue. *Gastroenterology* 1998;115:211.

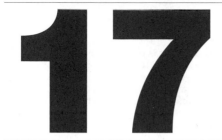

Colon Neoplasms

Eugene F. Yen

INTRODUCTION

Annually, there are 140,000 new cases and 55,000 deaths attributed to **colorectal cancer (CRC)**, the second leading cause of overall cancer-related mortality. The 5-yr survival rate for localized cancers is >90%, whereas the 5-yr survival for those with invasive cancer is <10%. Depending on the type of polyp found, the estimated time from adenoma to malignancy is 4–12 yrs, making screening a vital tool in the treatment and prevention of CRC.

Epidemiology

Epidemiologic data on the prevalence of GI polyps in asymptomatic patients vary from 23–41%. Prevalence of colon cancer is determined by two factors: age and the inherent risk in a certain population. Age is associated with not only a higher prevalence of polyps, but also multiple polyps, severe dysplasia, and larger adenoma size. Distribution of polyps has been found to be uniform throughout the colon. However, in patients >60 yrs, adenomas tend to be found more proximally.

Different populations also carry different risk, as this is seen most prominently in Hawaiian-Japanese people, who have a prevalence of adenoma as high as 50–60%. Conversely, Japanese people living in Japan have prevalence rates <12%. This disparity strongly implies that lifestyle and environmental factors also play a role in CRC. Also, in populations that consume a diet high in red meat and fat and low in fruits, vegetables, and fiber (United States, Canada, Australia, Western Europe), there is up to a 20-fold increase in mortality rates from CRC.

Risk factors include a family history of CRC, personal history of colon polyps or cancer, history of inflammatory bowel disease (IBD), and certain familial polyposis syndromes. Although there are well-described genetic polyposis syndromes, approximately 95% of adenomas and carcinomas arise sporadically. Dietary fiber, plant foods, and carbohydrates have been shown to have a protective benefit in preventing adenomas. In addition, cigarette smoking has been found to increase adenomas but not cancer risk. Patients are thus encouraged to eat a diet that is low in total fat and high in fruits, vegetables, and fiber to decrease the risk of developing adenomas and CRC. The Australian Polyp Prevention Trial found that after a 1- to 2-yr diet low in fat and high in fiber, recurrent adenomas were unchanged, but the frequency of large adenomas was reduced. Finally, although a relationship between dietary fat and CRC exists, there is no correlation between hyperlipidemia and CRC.

Clinical conditions that predispose to colon cancer include ureterosigmoidostomy and acromegaly. Ureterosigmoidostomy, a urinary diversion procedure in which the ureters are implanted into the sigmoid colon, is associated with an increased risk of colon cancer, usually >15 yrs after surgery. In addition, patients with *Streptococcus bovis* bacteremia frequently have underlying colon cancer and must undergo colonoscopy.

CAUSES

Pathophysiology

The earliest change in the progression of colon cancer is the adenoma, which consists of benign neoplastic epithelium. Adenomas are believed to result from a failure in the normal process of cell proliferation and apoptosis. Polyps arise in colonic crypts in which the proliferative component of the crypt, usually confined to the base, extends through the entire crypt. Histologically, the tubular adenoma is the most common subgroup, representing 80–86% of all adenomatous polyps. These lesions tend to be small and exhibit only mild dysplasia, seen microscopically as a complex network of branching adenomatous glands. Villous adenomas tend to have a higher degree of dysplasia, with adenomatous glands extending through to the center of the polyps, thereby appearing grossly as a finger-like projection.

It is widely accepted that **adenomatous polyps** lead to colon cancer. This is supported by several studies, including the National Polyp Study, which found that removal of adenomas resulted in a lower incidence of CRC. In confirmed colon cancers, residual adenomatous tissue can be found within cancerous tissue. Likewise, small foci of cancer can be found in adenomas, yet they are very rare in normal bowel. Surgical colon specimens with cancer also contain adenomatous polyps in one-third of cases, and polyps are also seen in two-thirds of colons with >1 cancerous lesion.

Increasingly, molecular studies suggest a series of somatic DNA mutations that must occur for a polyp to transform from adenoma to carcinoma. Among the earliest mutations is inactivation of the adenomatous polyposis coli (APC) gene. Other later changes include mutations of the K-ras protooncogene, DNA hypomethylation, 18q inactivation, and p53 (tumor suppressor gene) inactivation. The accumulation of abnormalities results in a stepwise progression over approximately 10 yrs from normal mucosa to adenoma to carcinoma. Detection of these mutations from sloughed cells in stool samples may eventually prove to be a useful screening test for early CRC.

PRESENTATION

Most patients with colonic polyps are asymptomatic but may occasionally present with occult or overt bleeding from the GI tract. Villous adenomas >3 cm have been found to cause a secretory diarrhea, which may lead to volume depletion and electrolyte abnormalities. Many adenocarcinomas are also asymptomatic but may present with certain symptoms depending on location. Right-sided cancers may grow large before producing any symptoms due to the larger caliber of the cecum and ascending colon. Often, iron-deficiency anemia is the only manifestation of right-sided cancer. Tumors in the left side of the colon may present with symptoms of obstruction earlier, including abdominal distention, bloating, and constipation. Rectal or sigmoid cancers often cause hematochezia, constipation, or thinning of the stools. Consequently, the new development of any of the symptoms, especially in older patients, mandates colonoscopic evaluation.

MANAGEMENT

Diagnostic Evaluation

Average-Risk Individuals
Screening for CRC involves evaluation of average-risk individuals and should begin at age 50 yrs. Until recently, various screening protocols were used, including yearly fecal occult blood testing, periodic flexible sigmoidoscopy, and air contrast barium enema. These tests were used in various combinations and generally showed a reduction in overall mortality, suggesting that screening for CRC is useful. Multiple studies have shown, however, that these screening protocols have limited sensitivity and specificity and may miss a substantial number of advanced neoplasms. In addition, patients who have a positive test eventually require colonoscopy for diagnosis and removal of adenomatous polyps. For those reasons, most groups now advocate colonoscopy as the screening procedure of choice for average-risk individuals. The

optimal interval for colonoscopic screening has not yet been determined, but at this point, repeating the test every 10 yrs seems most appropriate.

High-Risk Individuals
Surveillance for CRC should be performed in individuals at increased risk for CRC. High-risk groups include those with IBD, familial polyposis syndromes, and personal or family histories of CRC. These patients appear to benefit from colonoscopy for surveillance of CRC.

INFLAMMATORY BOWEL DISEASE. In patients with Crohn's colitis or ulcerative colitis, there is evidence that surveillance colonoscopy is effective in reducing the mortality from CRC. However, given that there is an increased risk of dysplasia with duration of disease, current recommendations are to perform surveillance colonoscopy every 1–3 yrs on patients with pancolitis for >8 yrs or left-sided colitis for >15 yrs. Patients with ulcerative colitis have polyps that are inflammatory in nature, but adenomas should be managed similarly to polyps in patients without ulcerative colitis. Patients should have random biopsies taken every 10 cm throughout the entire colon. The finding of high-grade dysplasia mandates colectomy, whereas low-grade dysplasia is more controversial, with many experts also recommending colectomy.

FAMILIAL POLYPOSIS SYNDROMES. Familial polyposis syndromes represent only 5% of all CRC cases. For patients with familial adenomatous polyposis (FAP) or Gardner's syndrome, annual sigmoidoscopy should begin at age 10–12 yrs. Because FAP patients have a 100% risk of developing CRC by age 40 yrs, patients should undergo colectomy as soon as polyposis is found or after puberty.

HEREDITARY NONPOLYPOSIS COLORECTAL CANCER. Also known as Lynch syndrome, hereditary nonpolyposis colorectal cancer (HNPCC) is an autosomal-dominant familial colon cancer with fewer polyps than seen in FAP. HNPCC is further divided into Lynch I and II, with the latter being associated with other cancers in the uterus, ovary, breast, stomach, and pancreas. The diagnosis is based on the Amsterdam Criteria (Table 17-1). An estimated 68–75% of patients with HNPCC develop CRC by the age of 65 yrs, with the average age at diagnosis being 45 yrs. In addition, the risk of endometrial carcinoma is 30–39% by age 70 yrs, as opposed to 3% in the general population. Surveillance colonoscopy for HNPCC should begin at age 20–25 yrs and be performed every 2 yrs until age 40 yrs, followed by annual screening thereafter. Screening should involve all members of a family who meet the Amsterdam Criteria. Genetic testing for germline mutations in DNA mismatch repair genes (MLH1 and MSH2) is also available. A different approach is to examine the cancerous colon tissue from a patient for microsatellite instability (MSI). MSI indicates frequent genetic mutations throughout the genome, a feature seen in nearly all cancers from HNPCC, as opposed to only approximately 15% in sporadic cases of colon cancer. If the MSI is positive, genetic testing should be performed. It is now encouraged that both Amsterdam Criteria–positive families and those with strong but Amsterdam Criteria–negative family histories undergo genetic counseling, MSI testing, and mutation testing.

FAMILY HISTORY. The overall colon cancer risk in those with multiple first-degree relatives or a single first-degree relative diagnosed before age 40 yrs is 3–4 times that of the general population. Screening colonoscopy should be performed for these patients at age 40 yrs or 10 yrs younger than the age of the youngest affected relative. The current recommended interval for screening is every 5 yrs. In patients with a single first-degree relative with CRC or adenoma diagnosed at age >60 yrs, their risk of developing CRC is

TABLE 17-1. AMSTERDAM CRITERIA FOR HEREDITARY NONPOLYPOSIS COLORECTAL CANCER

Three relatives with colon cancer, two of whom must be first-degree relatives of the third

Colon cancer in two consecutive generations

One case diagnosed before age 50 yrs

TABLE 17-2. COLONOSCOPIC SURVEILLANCE FOR COLORECTAL POLYPS

	Risk	Repeat colonoscopy
Single adenoma, <1 cm, low-grade dysplasia	Low	5 yrs
Multiple adenomas, ≥ 1 cm, villous architecture, high-grade dysplasia	Moderate	3 yrs
Malignant polyps, large sessile adenomas, multiple adenomas	High	6–12 mos
Hyperplastic polyps	None	10 yrs

increased to 2 times that of the general population. In addition, their risk for colon cancer is the same at age 40 yrs as the general population at age 50 yrs, so recommended screening should begin at age 40 yrs and continue at normal routine intervals.

PERSONAL HISTORY. The National Polyp Study provides the best evidence for surveillance colonoscopy after adenomatous polyp removal. In a cohort of 1418 patients, the group that underwent colonoscopic surveillance after adenomatous polyp removal had rates of CRC that were 76–90% lower compared to the control groups who had polypectomy but had not undergone surveillance. The recommended interval for repeat surveillance colonoscopy depends on the findings on the initial study. Table 17-2 lists the surveillance recommendations for patients with colorectal polyps.

TREATMENT

Adenomas

Most polyps found by flexible sigmoidoscopy or colonoscopy can be resected completely using electrocautery techniques. Current guidelines for treatment of adenomatous polyps include initial clearing of the colon by colonoscopy, followed by surveillance colonoscopy in 3 yrs for most patients. As discussed above, surveillance intervals should be based on the extent of polyps and the individual patient's family history. Individuals with hyperplastic polyps are not at increased risk for development of CRC, and colonoscopy every 10 yrs is sufficient.

Colorectal Cancer

For patients diagnosed with CRC, the treatment of choice is **surgical resection.** The goal of surgery is removal of the affected segment of bowel and lymphatic vessels, with the extent of resection determined by the distribution of blood vessels and lymphatic drainage. For patients with rectal cancers, surgical treatment depends on the location, size, and extent of involvement of the rectal tumors. Therapies include low anterior resection for upper rectal cancers and abdominoperineal resection for poorly differentiated cancers, large bulky tumors found deep in the pelvis, and cancers involving the lower rectum.

In patients with CRC, synchronous polyps can occur in 20–40% of cases. Preoperative colonoscopy is recommended in patients before undergoing resection. If the tumor is obstructing and cannot be traversed by the colonoscope, barium enema may be performed to evaluate the proximal colon. CRCs tend to metastasize to regional lymph nodes, liver, and lung. Thus, CT scanning is recommended for patients with an abnormal liver exam or liver enzymes, but whether routine CT should be performed for staging remains controversial. Anatomic staging of cancers occurs at the time of surgery, using the TNM (tumor, node, metastasis) universal system or a modification of the Dukes system for CRC (Table 17-3).

Staging can direct the clinician to assess a patient's postsurgical outcome and need for adjuvant therapy. Adjuvant chemotherapy with 5-fluorouracil and levamisole or leucovorin improves survival in patients with Dukes C colon cancer. For Dukes B and C rectal cancers, radiation therapy and adjuvant chemotherapy appear to decrease the

TABLE 17-3. DUKES MODIFIED (ASTER AND COLLER) STAGING SYSTEM FOR COLORECTAL CANCER

Stage	Criteria	Estimated 5-yr survival (%)
A	Invades submucosa	>90
B1	Invades muscularis, no penetration through bowel wall, negative nodes	85
B2	Penetrates bowel wall, negative nodes	70–75
C1	Invades muscularis, no penetration of bowel wall, positive nodes	35–65
C2	Penetrates bowel wall, positive nodes	35–65
D	Distant metastases	<5

rate of local pelvic occurrence. Follow-up colonoscopy should be performed at 3 yrs, with subsequent surveillance intervals determined by endoscopic findings. Patients with obstructing metastatic cancers should undergo palliative resection or endoscopic stenting to prevent complete obstruction.

POLYPOSIS STATES

Various polyposis states are recognized based on histopathology, familial inheritance, and distribution in the GI tract. Identification of mutations in the APC gene in the 5q21-q22 region has allowed clinicians to categorize familial polyposis syndromes and their variations.

Familial Adenomatous Polyposis

FAP is the most common inherited polyposis syndrome, with a prevalence of 1/5,000 to 1/7,500. It is an autosomal-dominant disease characterized by hundreds to thousands of adenomatous polyps in the large intestine, with a 100% progression to colon cancer if not resected. Patients with FAP usually report symptoms after puberty, with the average age for diagnosis at 36 yrs and death from cancer at 42 yrs. Despite this, the natural history of onset of polyposis to CRC is estimated to be 10–15 yrs. Screening known FAP gene carriers with yearly sigmoidoscopy has allowed clinicians to identify polyps in 50% of patients.

In addition to colonic polyps, patients with FAP also frequently have upper GI manifestations. Gastric polyps occur in 30–50% of cases, but most are nonneoplastic, characterized by hyperplasia of fundic glands without epithelial dysplasia. Duodenal adenomas occur in 60–90% of FAP patients, and the lifetime incidence of duodenal cancer is 4–12%, >100 times the risk of the normal population. Most duodenal adenomas involve the periampullary region and may obstruct the biliary system. Patients with a history of duodenal polyps should undergo yearly surveillance upper endoscopy.

Gardner's Syndrome

Gardner's syndrome is a less common variant of FAP and includes the same genetic lesions and GI manifestations as FAP. Gardner's variant is associated with additional extraintestinal features, such as osteomas in the mandible, skull, and long bones. In addition, >90% of Gardner's syndrome patients have congenital hypertrophy of the retinal pigmented epithelium (CHRPE), consisting of pigmented ocular fundus lesions. CHRPE is seen in only 5% of controls, so presence of such lesions bilaterally, especially in those with a family history, could serve as a reliable marker for gene carriage in adenomatous polyposis. Other abnormalities found in Gardner's syndrome include benign soft tissue tumors and tumors of the thyroid, adrenal gland, and hepatobiliary system. Another complication is the development of diffuse mesenteric fibromatosis, or desmoid tumors, which are found in 8–13% of patients with Gardner's syndrome. These tumors can cause GI obstruction or constriction of the mesenteric vasculature or ureters. The mechanism of the development of desmoid tumors is unclear, so there is no single approach proven to prevent or treat this condition, which ranks second behind metastatic disease among the lethal complications of polyposis syndromes. Despite their variable manifestations, FAP and Gardner's syndrome involve the same genetic locus, the APC gene, and no patterns of mutation exist to distinguish between the two syndromes.

Turcot's Syndrome

Turcot's syndrome, also known as *glioma-polyposis*, is a syndrome of familial polyposis with primary tumors of the CNS. APC mutations are found in these patients, but no association can be found between specific mutations and the development of brain tumors. CNS tumors found in Turcot's syndrome are of different histologic types, depending on the particular genetic mutation. Those with germline mutations of the APC gene tend to have medulloblastomas, whereas those with mutations in DNA base mismatch repair genes typically have glioblastoma multiforme tumors.

Attenuated Familial Adenomatous Polyposis

Attenuated FAP is a rare variant of FAP consisting of fewer colonic adenomas. These adenomas often have a flat rather than polypoid growth pattern and tend to cluster in the proximal colon. Also known as *hereditary flat adenoma syndrome*, this condition is more aptly termed *attenuated FAP* for the finding of germline mutations in the APC gene. Much like FAP, patients are prone to upper GI adenomas and fundic gland polyps, but CRCs tend to occur in patients at a later age (approximately 55 yrs).

Peutz-Jeghers Syndrome

Peutz-Jeghers syndrome is an autosomal-dominant disease consisting of mucocutaneous pigmentation and GI polyposis. Patients manifest mucocutaneous pigmentation in infancy and childhood, with melanin deposits around the nose, lips, hands, feet, and buccal mucosa. Lesions are green-black to brown and fade during puberty, with the exception of buccal lesions. Hamartomatous polyps can be found in the stomach, small intestine, and colon but most commonly appear in the small intestine. Polyps in Peutz-Jeghers are unique hamartomas characterized by glandular epithelium with an abnormal framework of smooth muscle that is contiguous with the muscularis mucosa.

Although hamartomas are not true neoplasms, these polyps may grow in size and cause bleeding, small bowel obstruction, or intussusception. Cancer in the small bowel or colon is seen with increased frequency in patients with Peutz-Jeghers syndrome. Also, benign polyps can be found in the nose, bronchi, bladder, gallbladder, and bile duct. In 5–12% of female patients with Peutz-Jeghers, ovarian cysts and ovarian sex chord tumors can be seen. Similarly, Sertoli cell testicular rumors can be seen in young boys, causing feminizing features. Management of patients with Peutz-Jeghers syndrome includes screening of potential family members with colonoscopy, upper GI series films to evaluate for small bowel polyps, and pelvic U/S for girls and physical exam of the genitalia in boys.

Juvenile Polyposis

Juvenile polyposis, an autosomal-dominant disorder, encompasses at least three different forms: familial juvenile polyposis coli, familial juvenile polyposis of the stomach, and generalized juvenile polyposis. Histologically, juvenile polyps are hamartomas, consisting of an excess of lamina propria and dilated cystic glands. Juvenile polyps are tumors of the mucosa rather than the epithelium, as seen in hyperplastic and adenomatous polyps.

Normally, these polyps are solitary and located in the rectums of children. There is an increased risk of colon cancer in these patients, arising in mixed juvenile adenomatous polyps or synchronous adenomatous polyps. Other complications include bleeding, obstruction, or intussusception in childhood, seen mostly in childhood as the polyps increase in size.

Management for potentially affected family members includes colonoscopy and careful histologic exam of polyps with adenomatous foci. Juvenile polyps should generally be removed because of their tendency to bleed or obstruct.

Cowden's Disease

Cowden's disease, or multiple hamartoma syndrome, is a rare autosomal-dominant disorder. It is characterized by multiple hamartomatous polyps and the presence of mucocutaneous lesions, including lichenoid and verrucous facial papules, acral keratoses, and oral papillomas. Other manifestations include breast lesions ranging from fibrocystic disease to breast cancer in 50% of patients and thyroid abnormalities, including cancer and multinodular goiter, seen in 10–15% of patients. However, polyps in the GI tract pose no increased risk for colon cancer, so clinical surveillance in patients with Cowden's disease is unnecessary.

Nonfamilial Polyposis Syndromes

Acquired polyposis syndromes also exist, with the differential diagnosis including inflammatory polyps (pseudopolyps), lymphomas, lipomas, hyperplastic polyps, and pneumatosis cystoides intestinalis. The most common nonneoplastic polyp is the hyperplastic polyp, which is made up of well-differentiated goblet and absorptive cells with orderly cell maturation. These polyps are usually small, averaging <5 mm. None of these conditions is associated with an increased risk of colon cancer.

KEY POINTS TO REMEMBER

- Annually, there are 140,000 new cases and 55,000 deaths attributed to CRC, the second leading cause of overall cancer-related mortality.
- Depending on the type of polyp found, the estimated time from adenoma to malignancy is 4–12 yrs, making screening a vital tool in the treatment and prevention of CRC.
- Risk factors for CRC include a family history of CRC or colon polyps, personal history of colon polyps or cancer, history of IBD, and certain familial polyposis syndromes.
- Patients with *Streptococcus bovis* bacteremia frequently have underlying colon cancer and must undergo colonoscopy.
- Periodic colonoscopy (most likely every 10 yrs) is the best screening test for individuals at average risk for CRC.
- Surveillance colonoscopy should be performed on patients with IBD who have had pancolitis for >8 yrs or left-sided colitis for >15 yrs.
- FAP patients have a 100% risk of developing CRC by age 40 yrs and should undergo colectomy as soon as polyposis is found or after puberty.
- Adjuvant chemotherapy with 5-fluorouracil and leucovorin is recommended for patients with Dukes C colon cancer. For Dukes B and C rectal cancers, radiation therapy and adjuvant chemotherapy appear to decrease the rate of local pelvic occurrence.

REFERENCES AND SUGGESTED READINGS

Burt RW. Impact on family history on screening surveillance. *Gastrointest Endosc* 1999;49:S41.

Correa P. Epidemiology of polyps and cancer. In: *The pathogenesis of colorectal cancer*. Philadelphia: WB Saunders, 1978:126.

Lieberman DA, Weiss DG, Bond JH, et al. Use of colonoscopy to screen asymptomatic adults for colorectal cancer. *N Engl J Med* 2000;343:162.

Muto T, Bussey HJR, Morson BC. The evolution of cancer of the colon and rectum. *Cancer* 1975;36:2251.

Rex DK, Johnson DA, Lieberman DA, et al. Colorectal cancer prevention 2000: screening recommendation of the American College of Gastroenterology. *Am J Gastroenterol* 2000;95:868.

Rhodes M, Bradbum DM. Overview of screening and management of familial adenomatous polyposis. *Gut* 1992;33:125.

Vogelstein B, Fearon ER, Hamilton S, et al. Genetic alterations during colorectal-tumor development. *N Engl J Med* 1988;319:525.

Winawer SJ, Fletcher RH, Miller RH, et al. Colorectal cancer screening: clinical guidelines and rationale. *Gastroenterology* 1997;112:594.

Winawer SJ, Fletcher RH, Rex D, et al. Colorectal cancer screening and surveillance: clinical guidelines and rationale. *Gastroenterology* 2003;124:544.

Winawer SJ, Zauber AG, Gerdes H, et al. Prevention of colorectal cancer by colonoscopic polypectomy. *N Engl J Med* 1993;329:1977.

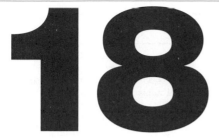

Inflammatory Bowel Disease

David S. Lotsoff

INTRODUCTION

Inflammatory bowel disease (IBD) is a spectrum of disorders characterized by varying types and degrees of intestinal inflammation. **Crohn's disease** and **ulcerative colitis (UC)** are the most common of the IBDs. These conditions are relatively common disorders that cause substantial morbidity. Because these diseases often affect a younger population, early diagnosis and intervention can often substantially improve quality of life and prevent complications.

Crohn's Disease

Crohn's disease is characterized by chronic transmural inflammation of the GI mucosa. The course is marked by exacerbations and remissions. In contrast to UC, the disease can affect any portion of the GI tract. The clinical course of Crohn's disease is often complicated by fistula formation, perianal disease, and strictures. The incidence (5/100,000) and prevalence (50/100,000) in the United States are similar to those in other industrialized countries. The disease affects all ages, but diagnosis is most commonly made in the second and third decade, with a second peak in incidence at age 60–80 yrs.

Ulcerative Colitis

UC is a chronic inflammatory disease of the colon and rectum characterized by a relapsing and remitting course. The rectal mucosa is almost invariably affected. On direct mucosal exam, shallow ulcerations and confluent inflammation are found to extend proximally from the anal margin. Bloody diarrhea is the predominant symptom and is more often seen in UC compared with Crohn's disease. Remission may be induced, but relapses are common, with the probability of relapse at 2 yrs being 80%. Men and women are affected equally, and the disease can present at any age. Extraintestinal symptoms may be seen in UC and may correlate or be unrelated to the timing of active colitis. The overall prognosis of UC is good, and there is no significant excess in mortality.

CAUSES

Crohn's Disease

The etiology of Crohn's disease is unknown, and the disease is neither medically nor surgically curable. Genetic studies suggest that Crohn's disease is a polygenic disorder. The current hypothesis proposes an excessive immune response in genetically susceptible individuals. Endogenous bacteria may possibly drive this response. Another hypothesis proposes that some cases of Crohn's disease may result from the interaction of environmental and genetic influences leading to impaired mucosal neutrophil function. The disease seems to be a twentieth-century phenomenon in industrialized countries given that the disease appears to be uncommon before Crohn's defining publication in 1932.

Factors that have been shown to exacerbate Crohn's disease include concomitant infection (both intestinal and extraintestinal), NSAID use, and smoking (in contrast

TABLE 18-1. COMPARISON BETWEEN CROHN'S DISEASE AND ULCERATIVE COLITIS

	Crohn's disease	Ulcerative colitis
Clinical findings	Abdominal pain, diarrhea, weight loss, vomiting, perianal disease, abdominal mass	Rectal bleeding, diarrhea
Endoscopy	Patchy involvement, rectal sparing, aphthous ulcers, ileal ulcers	Rectal involvement with continuous superficial ulceration
Radiology	Stricture, fistulas, terminal ileal disease (string sign)	Loss of haustra, continuous ulceration
Histology	Transmural disease, aphthous ulcers, granulomas	Abnormal crypt architecture, superficial inflammation

to UC, in which smoking seems to be protective). Although many patients and family members associate Crohn's exacerbations with stressful life situations, studies have not shown stress to correlate with the development of disease.

A role for enteric flora or an as yet identified fecal toxin in the pathogenesis of Crohn's disease is strongly suggested by the observation that fecal stream diversion from an involved segment of bowel attenuates the mucosal inflammation. Reestablishment of bowel continuity results in disease recurrence. Further evidence for a role of enteric flora is suggested by the effectiveness of antibiotics in the treatment of Crohn's disease.

Ulcerative Colitis

Like Crohn's disease, the etiology of UC remains unknown. In contrast to Crohn's disease, smoking seems to have beneficial effects in UC, with lower hospitalization rates in smokers compared to nonsmokers at the onset of UC. Low appendectomy rates have been reported in UC, but the significance of this finding is as yet undetermined. See Table 18-1 for a fuller comparison between ulcerative colitis and Crohn's disease.

PRESENTATION

Crohn's Disease

The diagnosis of Crohn's disease is made with a combination of clinical, endoscopic, pathologic, and radiographic findings.

Crohn's disease may present with GI symptoms, extraintestinal symptoms, or both. Symptoms include chronic diarrhea, abdominal pain, weight loss, fever, and rectal bleeding. Signs can include cachexia; abdominal tenderness or mass; or perianal fissures, fistulas, or abscess. The ileum and colon are the most commonly affected sites of intestinal involvement (Table 18-2). Gastric and duodenal manifestations may present with nausea and vomiting, epigastric pain, or gastric outlet obstruction. Common extraintestinal features are discussed later in this chapter. The extraintestinal complications can be independent of or parallel intestinal disease activity.

Ulcerative Colitis

The most common symptoms at presentation include rectal bleeding and tenesmus. Abdominal pain, usually related to defecation, is often localized to the left side. Diarrhea with blood and mucus and reports of fecal incontinence may be noted. Systemic symptoms may include fever, fatigue, and weight loss.

TABLE 18-2. PATTERNS OF CROHN'S DISEASE INVOLVEMENT

Gastroduodenitis	7%
Jejunoileitis	5%
Ileitis	28%
Ileocolitis	45%
Colitis	15%

MANAGEMENT

Diagnostic Evaluation

Crohn's Disease

Endoscopy is used to assess disease location, confirm the diagnosis of Crohn's disease, and obtain tissue for evaluation. Pathologic specimens can help to establish the diagnosis and differentiate between Crohn's disease and UC. Pathologic specimens in Crohn's disease show a chronic inflammatory infiltrate that spreads transmurally. Inflammation may be discontinuous with skip areas. Granulomas may also be present. As discussed below, mucosal biopsy is also used to screen for dysplasia or cancer.

Air contrast barium enema, small bowel follow through, or enteroclysis may be used to confirm the anatomic pattern of disease as well as evaluate for complications of the disease. CT scanning or MRI can be used to evaluate for the presence of intraabdominal abscesses and is useful in evaluating perianal complications.

Ulcerative Colitis

After infection has been excluded, the extent of inflammation should be established by endoscopy. Total colonoscopy may help to distinguish between Crohn's and UC, and biopsies from the entire colon and terminal ileum may be obtained. Alternatively, flexible sigmoidoscopy and double contrast barium enema may help to determine the extent of involvement. A barium enema can exacerbate the disease and should never be performed during an acute episode, especially if toxic megacolon or perforation is suspected. The extent and pattern of inflammation should be examined by endoscopy. Pathologic specimens show a diffuse chronic infiltrate confined to the mucosa, continuous disease, and cryptitis.

Treatment

Crohn's Disease

Management of Crohn's disease depends on disease location, severity, and any existing complications. Therapy may also be divided into induction therapy and maintenance therapy.

5-AMINOSALICYLIC ACID COMPOUNDS. Salicylates are used for induction of remission in mild to moderate active disease and have been suggested to be effective in reducing the risk of postop recurrence.

Sulfasalazine (3–6 g daily in divided doses) is a diazo-compound consisting of the sulfonamide sulfapyridine and 5-aminosalicylic acid (5-ASA). The azo bond is cleaved by colonic bacteria, releasing sulfapyridine and 5-ASA into the colon. The therapeutic effects are derived primarily from the 5-ASA moiety (mesalamine). This medication has considerable side effects (mostly due to its sulfa moiety). Nausea, vomiting, malaise, anorexia, and headache are dose related, whereas hypersensitivity reactions, such as rash, fever, hemolytic anemia, agranulocytosis, hepatitis, pancreatitis, and worsening of colitis, are idiosyncratic. Sulfasalazine is also ineffective in patients with small bowel involvement. It is, however, a reasonable choice in patients with arthritis or spondyloarthropathy because it is a disease-modifying antirheumatic drug.

Nonsulfa 5-ASA derivatives are better tolerated than sulfasalazine. Mesalamine (up to 4.8 g daily in divided doses) has been shown to facilitate steroid withdrawal after induction of remission, and it decreases the postop relapse rate. Because several types of release preparations are available, optimal use of 5-ASA preparations involves consideration of the site of disease involvement. Sustained-release preparations (e.g., Pentasa) should be used for small bowel involvement, whereas delayed-release preparations (e.g., Asacol) should be used for inflammation in the terminal ileum and colon.

CORTICOSTEROIDS. Corticosteroids may be used to induce remission. Both oral prednisone (40–60 mg daily) and IV methylprednisolone (40–60 mg daily) were found to induce remission in patients with active disease compared to placebo. Doses are typically tapered when a clinical response has been achieved due to the serious side effects of long-term steroid use. Approximately 50% of patients treated acutely with steroids become steroid dependent or refractory. Budesonide is a slow-release form of glucocorticoid with poor absorption that may take advantage of the first-pass effect in the liver with subsequent reduced systemic side effects. The role of corticosteroids for maintenance treatment is controversial. Most studies do not find a benefit using corticosteroids for maintenance of remission.

IMMUNOSUPPRESSIVE AGENTS. Oral azathioprine (2.5 mg/kg/day) and its metabolite 6-mercaptopurine (6-MP) (1.0–1.5 mg/kg/day) have been demonstrated to be effective in both induction and maintenance of remission in Crohn's disease. These agents are also effective for use as steroid-sparing agents and in fistulous disease and likely have a role in preventing postop relapses.

The use of azathioprine/6-MP also has disadvantages, such as a long onset of action and significant side effects. These medications take ≥ 2 mos, and sometimes ≥ 6 mos, to be effective. Agranulocytosis, pancreatitis, allergic reactions, hepatitis, and life-threatening infections have been reported. These side effects are reversible on discontinuation of therapy. The potential to cause secondary malignancies and the possibility of a teratogenic effect remain controversial issues. Some evidence suggests that monitoring for leukopenia serves as an indicator of effectiveness. However, if the leukocyte count falls to <3,000 cells/μL, leukopenia is regarded as severe, and azathioprine/6-MP should be stopped. CBCs should be monitored carefully on initiation of azathioprine/6-MP and, in the long term, should be checked at a minimum of every 3 mos because of the risk of delayed neutropenia. The necessary length of therapy for these drugs is also unclear, and one study suggests that the risk of relapse after 4 yrs of remission is similar whether the treatment was discontinued or maintained.

IV cyclosporine A in high doses (4 mg/kg/day) has been shown to be effective in severe fistulizing disease. Methotrexate (25 mg/wk SC or IM) has been shown to have benefit in chronically active Crohn's disease, and this agent may be of particular use in patients with joint or spine involvement. Current trials are investigating other immunosuppressants, such as tacrolimus and mycophenolate mofetil.

ANTIBIOTICS. Recent evidence suggests that the combination of metronidazole (250 mg PO qid) plus ciprofloxacin (500 mg PO bid) may be useful in the acute treatment of Crohn's disease. Metronidazole is the preferred antibiotic in those patients that suffer from fistulas or perianal disease, including abscesses. Antibiotics should also be considered in patients with bacterial overgrowth after bowel resection. Patients taking long-term metronidazole need to be monitored closely for the development of peripheral neuropathy, which can be irreversible. The onset of new neurologic symptoms mandates immediate discontinuation of metronidazole.

INFLIXIMAB. Infliximab (Remicade) is a chimeric anti–tumor necrosis factor monoclonal antibody that has been shown effective in refractory Crohn's disease. A placebo-controlled trial has shown infliximab (5 mg/kg at 0, 2, and 6 wks IV) to be beneficial in treating fistulas refractory to prior therapy with antibiotics, corticosteroids, or immunomodulatory agents. A follow-up study suggests a possible benefit in maintenance of remission on retreatment with infliximab every 8 wks.

Infliximab infusions have been associated with infusion reactions, particularly with repeat infusions given after prolonged intervals (>12 wks). Development of antichimeric and anti-DNA antibodies has also been reported. There have been reports of reactivation–of latent TB in patients treated with infliximab. Consequently, a purified protein–derivative skin test should be placed before therapy. Congestive heart failure has also been reported as an adverse effect. Other side effects are self-limited and mild and include headache, upper respiratory infection, and nausea. The long-term efficacy and safety profile of infliximab has not yet been determined.

ANTIDIARRHEAL AGENTS. Antidiarrheal agents, such as loperamide (Imodium) or codeine, may decrease the frequency and volume of diarrhea. Caution must be used to avoid toxic megacolon and infectious complications.

NUTRITIONAL THERAPY. Maintenance of adequate nutrition is essential in the therapy of Crohn's disease. Enteral nutrition is always favored over parenteral nutrition. Special consideration should be made in patients with a history of bowel resection or extensive small bowel involvement in regard to vitamin and nutrient supplementation. For example, patients with ileitis may need parenteral vitamin B_{12} supplementation. Osteopenia can be associated with Crohn's disease and, in some respects, may be related to concomitant steroid use.

Total parenteral nutrition with bowel rest may be an effective therapy alone or in combination with corticosteroids in refractory Crohn's disease, with remission rates up to 80%, but discontinuation of total parenteral nutrition leads to high relapse rates of 60% within 2 yrs.

SURGICAL MANAGEMENT. Surgical consultation is appropriate for patients with a tender abdominal mass, stricture, or obstruction. Abscesses require drainage under radiographic guidance or with surgical management.

Surgical resection is not curative in Crohn's disease. Surgical management is often necessary for complications of intractable hemorrhage, perforation, persistent obstruction, or abscess. Resection of involved mucosa is also used to manage severe disease refractory to medical management.

Suppurative perianal disease is often treated surgically with the placement of a noncutting seton. New therapeutic options for management of strictures include endoscopic balloon dilation and local injection of steroids. In addition, all strictures should be biopsied to exclude malignancy.

SCREENING FOR MALIGNANCY. Patients with Crohn's colitis have an estimated sixfold increase in risk of colonic adenocarcinoma compared to the general population. Patients with long-standing colitis or ileitis and patients who are <30 yrs at diagnosis are at an even higher risk. The average time from onset of Crohn's disease to diagnosis of cancer is approximately 16 yrs. It has been recommended that surveillance colonoscopy with mucosal biopsies be performed in patients with Crohn's disease every 3 yrs after 8 yrs of extensive colitis and after 15 yrs of distal colitis. Colectomy is recommended for high-grade dysplasia or cancer.

Ulcerative Colitis

Management of UC depends on extent of disease involvement and severity. Therapy may also be divided into induction therapy and maintenance therapy.

5-AMINOSALICYLIC ACID COMPOUNDS. Salicylates are used for induction of remission in mild to moderate active disease. Distal disease (proctitis) may be treated by local application of suppositories or enemas. Treatment of more extensive colitis consists of delayed 5-ASA preparations or sulfasalazine. Balsalazide (750 mg PO tid) is a colonic-release preparation that may be more effective and better tolerated than other 5-ASA preparations. Salicylates are also the mainstay of medical treatment to maintain remission in UC. 5-ASA derivatives are usually better tolerated than sulfasalazine due to the side effects associated with its sulfa moiety.

CORTICOSTEROIDS. Corticosteroids may also be used for mild to moderate active disease. Enemas or suppositories may be used to treat distal disease. Oral corticosteroids may also be considered for more extensive mild to moderate disease, especially if response to salicylates is slow or absent. Standard therapy of severe disease is traditionally based on the use of corticosteroids, either oral or IV. As with Crohn's disease, long-term steroid use should be avoided. There is no evidence that steroids are effective in maintaining remission in UC.

IMMUNOSUPPRESSIVE AGENTS. The slow onset of action of azathioprine and 6-MP makes them relatively unhelpful in treating an acute UC flare. Their onset of action requires ≥ 2 mos to be effective. Azathioprine and 6-MP have been shown to be helpful in inducing remission and as steroid-sparing agents in chronic active disease. IV cyclosporine (4 mg/kg/day) has been shown effective in fulminant UC, but side effects include grand mal seizures, opportunistic infection, or bowel perforation.

TABLE 18-3. EXTRAINTESTINAL MANIFESTATIONS OF INFLAMMATORY BOWEL DISEASE

Complication	Parallels intestinal disease
Peripheral arthropathy	Yes
Spondyloarthropathy (ankylosing spondylitis, sacroiliitis)	No
Osteoporosis (often steroid-induced)	No
Episcleritis or scleritis	Yes
Anterior uveitis	No
Pyoderma gangrenosum	Yes
Erythema nodosum	Yes
Primary sclerosing cholangitis (usually ulcerative colitis)	No
Gallstones (after ileal resection)	No
Nephrolithiasis (usually Crohn's disease)	No

ANTIDIARRHEAL AGENTS. Drugs such as loperamide, tincture of belladonna, tincture of opium, and codeine may be beneficial in decreasing diarrhea but are contraindicated in severe exacerbations of UC because of the risk of toxic megacolon.

SURGICAL MANAGEMENT. Total colectomy should be considered for acutely ill patients with systemic toxicity who do not respond to medical therapy within 48 hrs; thus, surgical consultation is advised. Proctocolectomy or colectomy with rectal preservation is curative in these patients, and the mortality of colectomy, even in severe cases, is low. Advances in surgical technique have allowed for the creation of an ileal reservoir or pouch with ileoanal anastomosis, and a permanent ileostomy is not required.

SCREENING FOR MALIGNANCY. Risk factors for malignancy include family history of colon cancer, long-standing disease of >8 yrs, disease extent proximal to the sigmoid colon, and sclerosing cholangitis. UC patients have a 20-fold increase in risk of the development of colorectal cancer compared with controls. Surveillance colonoscopy should be performed as for Crohn's colitis.

SPECIAL TOPICS IN INFLAMMATORY BOWEL DISEASE

Extraintestinal Manifestations

Complications outside the GI tract contribute considerable morbidity in the minority of patients that develop them. The extraintestinal manifestations may be independent of or parallel intestinal disease activity. Generally, those conditions that parallel disease activity should be treated with intensification of antiinflammatory medications. Other conditions are treated independent of intestinal disease. Table 18-3 lists the most common extraintestinal complications.

Microscopic Colitis

Microscopic colitis is comprised of two entities: collagenous colitis and lymphocytic colitis. They are diseases of unknown etiology and are relatively uncommon, although the number of reported cases continues to increase. These conditions are characterized by watery diarrhea, weight loss, abdominal pain, and nausea. In contrast to Crohn's disease and UC, endoscopic and radiographic studies are typically normal or nonspecific. Diagnosis is made only by histologic exam of colon biopsies. Consequently, all patients undergoing endoscopic evaluation for diarrhea should have random colonic biopsies taken. Mucosal specimens reveal a chronic inflammatory infiltrate in the lamina propria. Collagenous colitis is associated with a thickened subepithelial collagen layer. The disease course is benign and sometimes relapsing and remitting. A minority of patients respond to treatment with antidiarrheals and bulking agents. Case studies have reported success using sulfasalazine, 5-ASA preparations, corticosteroids, and metronidazole. A double-blind, placebo-controlled trial demonstrated the effectiveness of bismuth subsalicylate in the treatment of microscopic colitis (262 mg, 3 tablets PO tid).

KEY POINTS TO REMEMBER

* Ulcerative colitis is characterized by rectal involvement with continuous superficial ulceration and presents with diarrhea and rectal bleeding.
* Crohn's disease may involve any part of the GI tract from mouth to anus and more commonly presents with abdominal pain, diarrhea, or weight loss.
* Factors that have been shown to exacerbate Crohn's disease include concomitant infection, NSAID use, and smoking.
* The ileum and colon are the most commonly affected sites of intestinal involvement in Crohn's disease.
* 5-ASA compounds and corticosteroids are useful for inducing remission in mild to moderately active Crohn's disease.
* Long-term steroid use should be avoided in both Crohn's disease and UC. Azathioprine or 6-MP may be used as a steroid-sparing agent.
* Surgical resection is not curative in Crohn's disease. Surgical management is often necessary for complications of intractable hemorrhage, perforation, persistent obstruction, or abscess.
* Surveillance colonoscopy with mucosal biopsies should be performed in patients with Crohn's disease or UC every 3 yrs after 8 yrs of extensive colitis and after 15 yrs of distal colitis.
* Extraintestinal symptoms that correlate with the activity of the patient's colitis include peripheral arthritis, episcleritis, pyoderma gangrenosum, and erythema nodosum. Ankylosing spondylitis, anterior uveitis, and sclerosing cholangitis are unrelated to intestinal disease activity.

REFERENCES AND SUGGESTED READINGS

Ardizzone S, Molteni P, Bollani S, Bianchi Porro G. Guidelines for the treatment of ulcerative colitis in remission. *Eur J Gastroenterol Hepatol* 1997;9:836–841.

Brandt LJ, Bernstein LH, Boley SJ, Frank MS. Metronidazole therapy for perineal Crohn's disease: a follow-up study. *Gastroenterology* 1982;83:383–387.

Frizelle FA, Santoro GA, Pemberton JH. The management of perianal Crohn's disease. *Int J Colorectal Dis* 1996;11:227–237.

Greenstein AJ, Sachar DB, Smith H, et al. A comparison of cancer risk in Crohn's disease and ulcerative colitis. *Cancer* 1981;48:2742–2745.

Kirk AP, Lennard-Jones JE. Controlled trial of azathioprine in chronic ulcerative colitis. *BMJ* 1982;284:1291–1298.

Korelitz BI. Considerations of surveillance, dysplasia, and carcinoma of the colon in the management of ulcerative colitis and Crohn's disease. *Med Clin North Am* 1990;74:189–199.

Lichtinger S, Present DH, Kornbluth A, et al. Cyclosporine in severe ulcerative colitis refractory to steroid therapy. *N Engl J Med* 1994;330:1841–1845.

Marshall JK, Irvine EJ. Rectal aminosalicylate therapy for distal ulcerative colitis: a meta-analysis. *Ailment Pharmacol Ther* 1995;9:293–300.

Motley RJ, Rhodes J, Kay S, Morris TJ. Late presentation of ulcerative colitis in ex-smokers. *Int J Colorectal Dis* 1988;3:171–175.

Munkholm P, Langholz E, Davidsen M, et al. Frequency of glucocorticoid resistance and dependency in Crohn's disease. *Gut* 1994;35:360–362.

Prantera C, Zannoni F, Scribano ML, et al. An antibiotic regimen for the treatment of active Crohn's disease: a randomized, controlled clinical trial of metronidazole plus ciprofloxacin. *Am J Gastroenterol* 1996;91:328–332.

Present DH, Rutgeerts P, Targan S, et al. Infliximab for the treatment of fistulas in patients with Crohn's disease. *N Engl J Med* 1999;340:1398–1405.

Summers RW, Switz DM, Sessions JT Jr, et al. National Cooperative Crohn's Disease Study: results of drug treatment. *Gastroenterology* 1979;77:847–869.

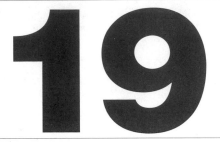

Irritable Bowel Syndrome

Clinton T. Snedegar

INTRODUCTION

Background

The functional GI disorders comprise chronic or recurrent conditions for which no organic etiology can be found but that cause considerable discomfort for the patient and contribute to a large portion of visits to both primary care physicians and gastroenterologists. They share a complicated interaction between abnormal GI motility, visceral hypersensitivity, altered CNS processing of peripheral stimuli, and psychosocial factors. Symptoms may arise from any section of the GI tract and may overlap. These functional syndromes are listed in Table 19-1. The prototypical and most common functional GI disorder is **irritable bowel syndrome (IBS).**

Epidemiology

IBS comprises a group of functional bowel disorders in which abdominal discomfort or pain is associated with defecation or a change in bowel habits. Depending on the criteria used, as many as 10–20% of adults may report symptoms consistent with IBS at any given time, but of that number, only approximately 15% of those affected actually seek medical attention. The condition more commonly affects women in a ratio of 3–4:1. IBS is frequently seen in medical practice, comprising 12% of the diagnoses made in primary care practices and 28% of those made by gastroenterologists. The cost to society is considerable, accounting for approximately 3 million physician visits and $8 billion in direct medical costs each year in the United States alone. Indirect costs in the form of work absenteeism may reach as high as $16 billion/yr. The absentee rate for IBS is similar to that seen for the common cold.

CAUSES

Pathophysiology

No single pathophysiologic abnormality has been found to adequately explain the manifestations of IBS. There is currently believed to be a complex interplay between abnormalities of intestinal motility, visceral hypersensitivity, GI tract inflammatory processes, interaction along the brain-gut axis, and psychosocial factors.

IBS is characterized by having an increased motility response to stressors, meals, and balloon inflation in the GI tract when compared to normal patients. However, these motor responses are not well correlated to symptoms and are alone insufficient to explain the patient's reported symptoms. IBS may result from sensitization of afferent neural pathways from the gut in such a way that normal intestinal stimuli induce pain. IBS patients have a lower pain threshold to balloon distention of the colon as compared to normals, but they have normal sensitivity to somatic stimuli.

Intestinal inflammation may play a role in the development of IBS. The question of persistent neuroimmune interactions after infectious gastroenteritis has been raised. For example, approximately one-third of patients with IBS report that symptoms began after an acute enteric infection. Ten to twenty-five percent of patients presenting with an acute enteric infection go on to develop IBS-like symptoms.

TABLE 19-1. THE FUNCTIONAL GASTROINTESTINAL DISORDERS

Esophageal disorders
  Globus
  Rumination syndrome
  Functional chest pain of presumed esophageal origin
  Functional heartburn
  Functional dysphagia
Gastroduodenal disorders
  Ulcer-like dyspepsia
  Dysmotility-like dyspepsia
  Aerophagia
  Functional vomiting
Bowel disorders
  Irritable bowel syndrome
  Functional abdominal bloating
  Functional constipation
  Functional diarrhea
Functional abdominal pain
Functional disorders of the biliary tract and pancreas
  Gallbladder dysfunction
  Sphincter of Oddi dysfunction
Anorectal disorders
  Functional fecal incontinence
  Functional anorectal pain
  Pelvic floor dyssynergia

Brain-gut interactions play a large role in the manifestations of IBS. Current belief is that there exists some disconnect or imbalance between the higher modulatory centers and the peripheral motor and sensory pathways of the GI tract. As such, these connections are the focus of intense research and the target of therapies. Psychosocial factors are important in this interplay but not crucial in pathogenesis. Painful or pleasurable stimuli, strong emotion, and day-to-day experiences modify how visceral sensation is perceived. Psychological stress is known to exacerbate GI symptoms, and the patient's psychological framework modifies illness behaviors, such as seeking health care.

Classification

There are several different diagnostic criteria for IBS, but the most commonly cited are the **Manning and Rome criteria.** Manning originally devised his criteria in 1978 using an outpatient questionnaire evaluating patients with IBS and those with organic disease. The Manning criteria can be found in Table 19-2. The Rome II criteria are the most recent and encompassing criteria, asserted primarily as a tool for devising clinical studies in the area. The Rome II criteria can be found in Table 19-3. Although they are not necessary for diagnosis using the Rome II criteria, there are several supporting symptoms that help to solidify the diagnosis and further characterize the disorder into diarrhea-predominant, constipation-predominant, or mixed disease (Table 19-4).

TABLE 19-2.   THE MANNING CRITERIA

Pain eased after bowel movement	Abdominal distention
Looser stools at onset of pain	Mucus per rectum
More frequent bowel movements at onset of pain	Feeling of incomplete emptying

PRESENTATION
History and Physical Exam

Description of symptoms alone poorly specifies the disease regardless of the criteria used. IBS is a diagnosis that should be made after organic causes have been excluded, so a careful search for alarm symptoms should be done. Important alarm symptoms include weight loss, fever, persistent diarrhea, rectal bleeding, nocturnal pain and bowel changes, age >50 yrs, and family history of GI malignancy, inflammatory bowel disease, or celiac sprue. In addition, a short history of rapidly progressive symptoms suggests organic disease.

Likewise, the physical exam should be focused to exclude organic disease. Abdominal tenderness is commonly present due to the heightened visceral sensitivity noted in this population. Physical exam alarm signs include the presence of ascites, jaundice, organomegaly, abdominal mass, adenopathy, heme-positive stool, or neuropathy.

MANAGEMENT
Diagnostic Evaluation

Lab and invasive testing should be kept to a minimum. Although specificity of diagnosis is increased by using limited testing to rule out organic disease, extensive or repetitive investigations may serve only to reinforce illness behavior. Initial lab testing should include a complete metabolic profile, CBC, TSH test, and perhaps ESR. Stool analysis for culture, *Clostridium difficile*, and ova and parasites should be performed if diarrhea is the predominant symptom.

Endoscopy may be unnecessary in young patients presenting with classic features of IBS. Usually, flexible sigmoidoscopy is recommended to rule out inflammation or tumors in patients <40 yrs. Advantages to this approach include the ability to identify melanosis coli indicative of laxative abuse. Some investigators also note that endoscopic insufflation of the colon may allow detection of hypersensitivity to visceral pain. Colonoscopy is indicated in all patients >40 yrs or if inflammatory bowel disease is suspected in younger patients.

Treatment

There is a 30–80% placebo response rate in patients with IBS. Consequently, the most important components of treatment are patient education and reassurance while establishing a therapeutic relationship. The strength of the physician's relationship

TABLE 19-3.   THE ROME II CRITERIA

At least 12 wks, which need not be consecutive, in the preceding 12 mos of abdominal discomfort or pain that has two out of three features:

1. Relieved with defecation; and/or
2. Onset associated with a change in frequency of stools; and/or
3. Onset associated with a change in form (appearance) of stool

TABLE 19-4. SUPPORTIVE SYMPTOMS OF IRRITABLE BOWEL SYNDROME

Abnormal stool frequency (*abnormal* defined >3 bowel movements/day or <3 bowel movements/wk)

Abnormal stool form (lumpy/hard or loose/watery stool)

Abnormal stool passage (straining, urgency, or feeling of incomplete evacuation)

Passage of mucus

Bloating or feeling of abdominal distention

with the patient correlates to higher rates of patient satisfaction and fewer return visits. Table 19-5 identifies general management principles for patients with IBS or other functional bowel disorders.

The approach to therapy in IBS is multifaceted and should be tailored to the individual patient given the constellation and severity of symptoms. Current approaches include modification of **diet, psychosocial therapy,** and **drug therapy.**

Generally, increasing the amount of dietary fiber is recommended, particularly in those with constipation as the predominant symptom; this can be supplemented with natural fiber sources, such as psyllium, or synthetic fiber, such as methylcellulose. In patients who complain of bloating or gas, fiber supplementation may be associated with an increase in those symptoms. In that same population, exclusion of flatulogenic foods should be encouraged. These foods include beans, onions, celery, carrots, raisins, apricots, prunes, brussel sprouts, wheat germ, pretzels, and bagels.

Behavioral therapy may be useful in patients who correlate an increase in severity of symptoms with life stressors. Although response is sporadic, factors favoring a good response include high patient motivation, diarrhea or pain as the predominant symptom, overt psychiatric symptoms, and intermittent pain exacerbated by stress.

Although medical therapy is available and new drugs are currently in development, IBS is a lifelong condition with exacerbations and remittances, and medications should be minimized to the extent possible. Given the nonorganic nature of IBS, trials of medications are frequently part of the diagnostic process. These trials should be pursued for ≥ 4 wks before moving on to different therapy. Also, if a drug from one class fails, the patient may respond to a different drug in the same class.

The most frequently prescribed drugs in the treatment of IBS are the anticholinergic/antispasmodic agents. The only drugs of this class available in the United States are hyoscyamine (Levsin), 0.125–0.25 mg PO/SL q4h prn, and dicyclomine (Bentyl), 10–20 mg PO/IM q6h prn. These agents are most useful in patients with postprandial symptoms of abdominal pain, gas, bloating, or fecal urgency. They should be prescribed in such a way as to head off symptoms before their initiation, such as before meals.

Antidepressant medications are most useful in patients with chronic, refractory symptoms and are particularly helpful with those who have concurrent depressive

TABLE 19-5. GENERAL APPROACH TO IRRITABLE BOWEL SYNDROME AND THE FUNCTIONAL BOWEL DISORDERS

Minimize invasive testing, targeted to exclude other disorders

Avoid repetitive testing unless necessary

Determine patient expectations and goals

Education and reassurance with emphasis on benign nature of condition

Dietary modifications and fiber supplementation are first-line therapy

Reserve medications for difficult cases

Behavioral or psychological interventions for refractory irritable bowel syndrome and anxiety disorders. Some of the medications in this class have been found to be beneficial in neuropathic pain. Although the mechanism of action in IBS is unclear, it is thought that antidepressants act in some way to interrupt or modulate the interactions of the brain-gut axis. TCAs are usually used in low doses, much lower than those used in depression. A typical starting dose for nortriptyline or amitriptyline is 10–25 mg PO qhs. The anticholinergic properties of TCAs are particularly useful in diarrhea-predominant IBS. SSRIs are also being increasingly used, although experience in IBS is limited. One of the recognized side effects of SSRIs is diarrhea; as such, this agent may be more useful in constipation-predominant disease.

New agents in development are the serotonin modulators. Serotonin is a major GI tract neurotransmitter, and studies indicate that postprandial levels of serotonin in diarrhea-predominant IBS are significantly higher than in controls. Alosetron (Lotronex), a selective 5-hydroxytryptamine-3 receptor antagonist, was approved for treatment of women with diarrhea-predominant IBS but was subsequently withdrawn from the market after several cases of ischemic colitis were reported. Tegaserod (Zelnorm), 16 mg PO bid, is a 5-hydroxytryptamine-4 receptor agonist that exerts GI stimulatory effects and is indicated for short-term treatment of women with constipation-predominant symptoms.

KEY POINTS TO REMEMBER

- IBS comprises a group of functional bowel disorders in which abdominal discomfort or pain is associated with defecation or a change in bowel habits.
- The Manning and Rome II criteria help to separate functional from organic disease, and the history, physical, and limited lab and invasive testing increase the specificity of the diagnosis.
- There is a very high placebo response rate in treatment of IBS.
- The most important components of therapy are patient education and reassurance and establishment of a therapeutic physician–patient relationship.
- Dietary and supplemental fiber are generally recommended, although these may increase symptoms of bloating and gas in some patients.
- TCAs in low dose and SSRIs may be helpful in interrupting the abnormal interactions of the brain-gut axis.
- New therapies on the horizon focus on neuropeptides in the GI tract and CNS, particularly serotonin and its receptors.

REFERENCES AND SUGGESTED READINGS

Camilleri M. Management of the irritable bowel syndrome. *Gastroenterology* 2001; 120:652–668.

Drossman DA, Corazziari E, Tally NJ, et al., eds. *Rome II: the functional gastrointestinal disorders. Diagnosis, pathophysiology and treatment: a multinational consensus*, 2nd ed. McLean, VA: Degnon Associates, 2000.

Shen B, Soffer E. The challenge of the irritable bowel syndrome: creating an alliance between patient and physician. *Cleve Clin J Med* 2001;68(3):224–235.

Talley NJ, Colin-Jones D, Koch KL, et al. Functional dyspepsia: a classification with guidelines for diagnostic management. *Gastroenterol Int* 1991;4:145–160.

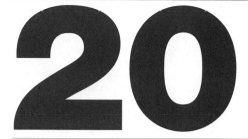

Acute Liver Disease

Clinton T. Snedegar

INTRODUCTION

Acute liver disease is a common cause of morbidity and mortality worldwide. Severity of disease can range from subclinical hepatitis with transient elevations of amino-transferase levels to fulminant hepatic failure and death. This chapter discusses the common causes of acute liver disease, including the viral hepatitides, liver abscesses, and drug- and toxin-mediated liver disease, and concludes with a discussion of acute liver failure.

VIRAL HEPATITIS

Hepatitis A

Of those cases of acute liver disease with a discernible etiology, the hepatitis A virus (HAV) is the most common cause worldwide but is a relatively uncommon cause in the United States. The virus is spread via the fecal–oral route; thus, in the United States, most outbreaks are associated with contamination of food by food-service workers. Disease severity may range from subclinical infection to, in rare instances, acute liver failure. The severity of disease is, in general, proportionate to the age at onset. Adults are more likely to have clinically evident disease than are children. Onset of jaundice is predated by a prodrome of constitutional symptoms, notably malaise, nausea, vomiting, abdominal pain, and fever. This prodrome may last for up to 1 wk and generally begins to resolve by the onset of jaundice, which may last for as long as 2 wks. Exam may reveal tender hepatomegaly, splenomegaly, or lymphadenopathy.

Aminotransferase levels increase during the prodromal phase, are usually >500, and rarely exceed 5000. Both direct and indirect bilirubin are elevated but usually to <25 mg/dL. Alkaline phosphatase is mildly elevated. Detecting serum antibodies against HAV makes the definitive diagnosis. Anti-HAV IgM is detectable in the acute phase of disease. Anti-HAV IgG is present in patients who have been exposed to the virus in the past. Management is conservative and should be directed at alleviating symptoms. Some patients may rarely require brief hospitalization for the purpose of IV fluids and parenteral antiemetics. There is no chronic liver disease associated with HAV.

Hepatitis B

Infection with the hepatitis B virus (HBV) is a common cause of both acute and chronic liver disease. In endemic areas such as Asia, the predominant mode of trans-mission is vertical. In most Western countries, the major routes of transmission are through unprotected sexual intercourse and injection drug use. Given the ease of test-ing for HBsAg, the risk of transfusion-related hepatitis due to HBV is quite low. Health care workers are at a slightly increased risk given exposure to patients with HBV through skin breaks and accidental needle sticks.

Hepatocyte necrosis in HBV infection is not believed to be secondary to the virus itself but rather due to the immune response to infection. It is believed that cytotoxic

T cells mediate lysis of infected hepatocytes. A fulminant course may be secondary to particularly aggressive immune clearance. The clinical manifestations of HBV infection are protean. Of all patients infected with the virus, only 30% become jaundiced. The incidence of acute liver failure is estimated at 1/200 to 1/1000 infected patients. Patients generally suffer constitutional symptoms, with resolution of these symptoms as jaundice develops. ALT levels commonly reach the low thousands, and serum ALT is usually greater than AST. If the ALT remains elevated for >6 mos, the patient has chronic disease.

Definitive diagnosis is made through testing for HBV-related antigens and antibodies.

- HBsAg is the hallmark of infection and is detectable 2–6 wks before the onset of symptoms. Persistent elevation beyond 6 mos indicates chronic infection.
- Anti-HBs is detected in patients who have recovered from infection or who have been vaccinated.
- Anti-HBc IgM is the first antibody to develop in acute HBV.
- Anti-HBc IgG is found in combination with anti-HBs in patients with past infection and with HBsAg in those with chronic infection.
- HBcAg (core antigen) is intracellular and cannot be detected in serum.
- HBeAg (early antigen) is a marker of active viral replication. It is positive concurrently with serum HBV DNA by PCR.
- A small number of people without HBeAg have active replication and detectable HBV DNA. These patients have a strain of virus called the *precore mutant*, in which a stop codon in the precore RNA prevents production of the HBeAg, but the pregenomic RNA is still translated into HBcAg, and replication is unaffected.

Treatment of acute HBV is largely supportive. Hospitalization is only required if dehydration occurs because of severe nausea and vomiting or if acute liver failure (<1%) develops. 1–5% of adults develop chronic HBV infection. Prevention is the best approach to acute HBV. The HBV vaccine is very effective and should be given to all infants and certain high-risk groups (health care workers, household contacts of HBV carriers, IV drug users, homosexual men, hemodialysis recipients). Postexposure prophylaxis with HBV vaccine and HBV immune globulin should be given with known exposures in previously unvaccinated individuals. (See also Chap. 21, Chronic Liver Disease.)

Hepatitis C

Chronic hepatitis C virus (HCV) is one of the main causes of chronic liver disease and the most common indication for liver transplantation in the United States. However, the acute phase of the disease often goes unrecognized, as <15% of patients have icteric hepatitis. It is known to be parenterally transmitted, but a large number of cases have no known method of acquisition. The acute phase is usually mild and occurs 6–12 wks after transmission. Fulminant hepatic failure is rare but can be seen in patients subsequently infected with HAV, making vaccination imperative. The diagnosis is made via the serum anti-HCV antibody or HCV RNA. HCV RNA becomes detectable within a few weeks of exposure. Experimental therapy with interferon with or without ribavirin is very effective in preventing chronic HCV. However, because most cases of acute HCV are undiagnosed, very few patients receive treatment for acute HCV. There is no effective vaccine against HCV. Up to 85% of patients eventually develop chronic HCV. (See also Chap. 21, Chronic Liver Disease.)

Hepatitis D

The hepatitis D virus (HDV), or delta agent, is dependent on HBV for infection. HDV may be acquired along with HBV, termed *coinfection*, or in a patient with established HBV, called *superinfection*. In coinfection, the clinical picture is that of acute HBV and is usually self-limited. Superinfection may present with acute hepatitis in a patient known to have chronic HBV or in an unrecognized carrier. The diagnosis is made via the anti-HDV antibody.

Hepatitis E

Hepatitis E virus (HEV) is similar to HAV in its route of transmission and clinical course. Aside from causing usually mild, self-limited icteric hepatitis, its primary clinical consequence is a highly fulminant course and association with mortality in pregnant women, particularly those in the second and third trimesters. This association is not well understood. Anti-HEV IgM is a good marker of recent infection.

Other Viruses

Other viruses implicated in acute liver disease, particularly in the immunocompromised population, include CMV, Epstein-Barr virus, human herpes virus, and VZV.

LIVER ABSCESSES

Pyogenic liver abscesses are most commonly associated with diseases of the biliary tract, such as cholangitis or biliary stones. However, other sources for bacterial infestation can occur, as bacteria can enter the liver via both the hepatic arterial or portal venous circulations. The most common organism found in pyogenic liver abscesses is *Escherichia coli*. Other enteric organisms are also frequently seen. Abscesses are most frequently located in the right lobe. They can be solitary or multiple, with multiple abscesses most common in cholangitis or systemic bacteremia. The typical presentation is fever and right upper quadrant abdominal pain. Jaundice may be present. Lab evaluation is significant for leukocytosis with liver enzyme abnormalities. Blood cultures are positive in most cases. If abscess is suspected, CT scanning is the most effective imaging study. A liver abscess should be aspirated if the organism is not identified on blood culture or if it is resistant to therapy. Empiric antibiotic therapy with ampicillin, gentamicin, and metronidazole (Flagyl) is recommended until the organism is identified. Abscesses not treated are fatal. Even with aspiration and antibiotic therapy, mortality reaches 10–25%.

Amebic abscesses, caused by *Entamoeba histolytica*, are common in tropical countries but relatively rare in the United States. In this disease, the amebic cyst is orally ingested and, in its life cycle, travels to the proximal colon, where it invades the colonic wall and travels to the liver via the portal circulation. There, it takes up residence, forming abscesses. Fever and right upper quadrant pain are the most common complaints. A history of travel to an endemic area can usually be obtained. ELISA or hemagglutinin assays of the blood can make the diagnosis. Aspirate of an amebic cyst is usually free of leukocytes. Therapy is metronidazole, 750 mg tid for 7–10 days.

Other, less common causes of liver infections are hydatid cysts (caused by the parasite *Echinococcus*), TB, leptospirosis, ascariasis, schistosomiasis, and the liver fluke.

HEPATOTOXIC AGENTS

There are a number of pharmacologic agents capable of producing acute hepatitis in either a dose dependent or idiosyncratic fashion. A list of common drugs implicated in acute liver disease can be found in Table 20-1. In practice, the two most clinically significant toxic agents are alcohol and acetaminophen.

Alcohol

Alcohol can cause a wide spectrum of liver disease, from fatty infiltration to chronic liver disease to alcoholic hepatitis and death. (See also Chap. 21, Chronic Liver Disease.) Heavy alcohol intake may induce a severe hepatitis with a 15–50% mortality rate. It is unclear why some alcoholics get acute disease, although those that do often have underlying cirrhosis. It appears that alcohol may induce an inflammatory cascade that is self-perpetuating and is not resolved once alcohol intake is stopped. The

TABLE 20-1. COMMON DRUGS IMPLICATED IN ACUTE LIVER DISEASE

Acetaminophen	Methotrexate
Allopurinol	Methyldopa
Amiodarone	Nitrofurantoin
Azathioprine	NSAIDs
Chlorpromazine	Penicillins
Dantrolene	Phenytoin
Fluoroquinolones	Tetracycline
Halothane	TMP-SMX
Isoniazid	Valproate
Ketoconazole	

clinical scenario is that of sudden jaundice, often with nausea, vomiting, or diarrhea, in a patient with a history of alcohol abuse. Ascites, encephalopathy, and coagulopathy may be present. Hepatomegaly and right upper quadrant tenderness are frequently noted on physical exam. Transaminases are elevated but usually not more than five times the upper limit of normal. The ratio of AST:ALT is usually >2:1. The best indicator of disease severity and prognosis is Maddrey discriminant function.

$$\text{Discriminant function} =$$
$$4.6 \times \text{PT prolongation time (secs)} + \text{bilirubin (mg/dL)}$$

A score of >32 carries a poor prognosis. Death is usually secondary to sepsis and multiorgan failure or upper GI hemorrhage. Therapy is primarily supportive. In milder disease with a discriminant function of <32, no specific intervention other than symptom relief is warranted. In those with severe disease, a number of interventions have been proposed, none of which has definitively shown to be of benefit. The most intensely studied agents have been corticosteroids, with studies showing variable response rates. Overall steroids are best avoided in cases of alcoholic hepatitis complicated by sepsis and GI hemorrhage.

Acetaminophen

The prevalence and ease of access to acetaminophen make it a commonly encountered cause of acute liver disease. Purposeful acetaminophen overdose may lead to acute liver failure, and it is the most common cause of acute liver failure in the United Kingdom. However, significant toxicity can also be seen in patients taking high therapeutic doses of acetaminophen in combination with alcohol, with ingestion of other medicines that induce the cytochrome P450 system, or in those with preexisting liver disease. Generally, in a patient without complicating factors, 15 g of acetaminophen is necessary to cause clinically significant hepatotoxicity in an adult. In overdose, the glucuronide and sulfate conjugating systems become saturated, leading to more acetaminophen being metabolized via the cytochrome P450 pathway. Toxic intermediates are formed, binding to hepatocellular proteins and leading to necrosis.

Clinically, in patients ingesting toxic doses of acetaminophen, symptoms of nausea, vomiting, and anorexia occur within 6 hrs of ingestion. Symptoms generally decline over the next several hours, but within 24–48 hrs, elevated transaminases, PT, and jaundice develop. Transaminases peak at 48–96 hrs and may frequently reach high into the thousands. A small percentage may go on to encephalopathy and acute liver failure. Acetaminophen levels should be drawn ≥ 4 hrs after ingestion and plotted on the Rumack-Matthews nomogram (Fig. 20-1). For patients fall-

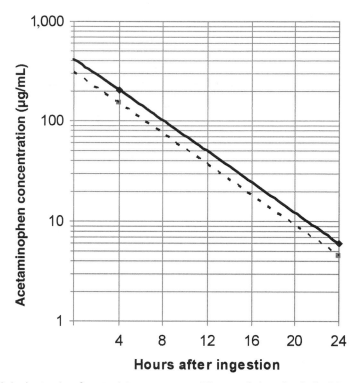

FIG. 20-1. Acetaminophen toxicity nomogram. The area below the dashed line represents nontoxic ingestion. The area between the two lines is potentially toxic, and the area above the solid line is likely to be toxic. Treatment should be initiated for any level above the dashed line. (Adapted from Rumack BH, Matthews H. Acetaminophen poisoning. *Pediatrics* 1975;55:871–876.)

ing into the potentially toxic range (above the dashed line), *N*-acetylcysteine (NAC) should be initiated. NAC provides a sulfhydryl group, which binds the free radical toxic intermediary and thus reduces liver damage. NAC should be given within 24 hrs of ingestion, with a loading dose of 140 mg/kg followed by 70 mg/kg every 4 hrs for a total of 17 doses. For patients with nausea and vomiting who cannot tolerate the foul-smelling oral solution, an IV preparation is now available in the United States. Although most cases of hepatotoxicity secondary to acetaminophen ingestion resolve with supportive care and have no long-term clinical sequelae, a small subset of patients develops fulminant hepatic failure leading to either death or transplantation.

ACUTE LIVER FAILURE

Acute liver failure is the presence of encephalopathy, coagulopathy, and jaundice in the setting of an acute liver insult. The most common known etiologies are viral hepatitis and hepatotoxic drugs, although in many cases, a distinct etiology cannot be found. Classification is based on encephalopathy, and onset of jaundice is described as follows:

- Hyperacute: encephalopathy within 7 days of onset of jaundice

- Acute: interval of 8–28 days from jaundice to encephalopathy
- Subacute: encephalopathy 5–12 wks after onset of jaundice

Overall, acute and subacute patients have a poorer prognosis. Acute liver failure carries a high mortality rate, and death is usually from associated complications, such as cerebral edema, renal failure, sepsis, and vascular collapse with multisystem organ failure. Except for specific causes of liver failure, such as acetaminophen overdose in which known treatment is available, therapy for acute liver failure is generally limited to supportive measures. The primary clinical manifestations and therapeutic options are as follows.

Hepatic encephalopathy is graded on a scale of I–IV (see Chap. 22, Cirrhosis). Patients with grade I may note mental slowness and a change in sleep patterns. Patients with grade IV are lethargic and may not respond to sternal rub. Asterixis is usually present, although in grade IV, it may be difficult to elicit the finding. The cause of encephalopathy is not well understood, but it is believed to be secondary to poor clearance of toxic metabolites by the damaged liver. The serum ammonia level is often used as a marker for encephalopathy, although it is an insensitive one, and assessment of encephalopathy should be guided by clinical judgment. Generally, CNS depressants should be avoided. Lactulose is the therapeutic agent of choice and may be given through a nasogastric tube if necessary. Oral antibiotics such as neomycin may also be useful. Although useful in treating mild encephalopathy, mortality is not improved with the use of these agents.

Cerebral edema and **intracranial HTN** are complications of grade IV encephalopathy but not a direct result. Etiology is not known. In its early phases, surges in ICP may be associated with external stimuli. In compensatory response, the patient's mean arterial pressure also rises. Herniation may occur. Alternatively, cerebral perfusion pressure may decrease to the point at which irreversible hypoxic brain injury ensues. CT scanning is not helpful in diagnosis. ICP monitors may be used, but parameters for their use are not clear. The osmotic diuretic mannitol may be used to lower the ICP, although caution should be exercised in cases of renal insufficiency. There is no role for parenteral steroids. The head of the bed should be elevated to 30 degrees, and unnecessary stimulation should be avoided. Hyperventilation using a mechanical ventilator may be helpful in the acute setting.

Hyperventilation is commonly seen, and may be multifactorial, from response to increased ICP, acidosis, or aspiration and pulmonary edema.

Hemodynamic changes of acute liver failure are similar to those seen in sepsis, with a high cardiac output and a low systemic vascular resistance. Assessment of the hemodynamic status is extremely difficult, particularly when renal failure is present, and pulmonary artery catheter monitoring is often helpful in management. Vasopressors such as norepinephrine may be required.

Renal failure is common and carries a very poor prognosis. It is usually multifactorial in origin, with poor perfusion from septic shock or volume depletion and from concomitantly toxic agents to both kidney and liver. Maintenance of renal perfusion and avoidance of nephrotoxic agents are imperative. If all reversible causes of renal failure have been addressed and renal failure persists, then the patient likely has an acute form of the hepatorenal syndrome. This carries a very poor prognosis. However, if the patient survives to transplantation, renal function usually returns to normal.

Hypoglycemia is frequently seen due to poor hepatic glucose production and consumption of glycogen stores and may be refractory to intravenous dextrose. Regular blood glucose monitoring should be performed.

Acid–base disturbances may be seen, especially metabolic acidosis in acetaminophen overdose, lactic acidosis, or renal failure, or alkalosis secondary to hyperventilation. Hypophosphatemia and hypomagnesemia are also frequently seen.

Coagulopathy is secondary to poor synthesis of clotting factors, particularly factor VII, leading to an elevated PT. Patients with severe liver failure often do not respond to vitamin K, although it should be attempted, at a dose of 10 mg SC daily for 3 days. FFP should be used for episodes of bleeding or before invasive procedures.

TABLE 20-2. THE KING'S COLLEGE CRITERIA INDICATING POOR PROGNOSIS

Acetaminophen-induced liver failure
  Arterial pH <7.30 or all three of the following concomitantly:
    PT >100 secs
    Creatinine >2.3 mg/dL
    Grade III–IV encephalopathy
Non–acetaminophen-induced liver failure
  PT >100 secs or any three of the following:
    Unfavorable etiology (seronegative hepatitis or drug reaction)
    Age <10 or >40 yrs
    Acute or subacute onset
    Serum bilirubin >17.6 mg/dL
    PT >50 secs

Infection is a common cause of death and is commonly seen because of the impaired reticuloendothelial system, decreased opsonization, and the frequent need for indwelling catheters and tracheal intubation. A high index of suspicion for infection is critical, with appropriate use of tissue culture and empiric antibiotic therapy as necessary.

Prognosis is strongly associated with grade of encephalopathy and varies with the cause of liver failure. Several criteria have been proposed for patients with severe liver failure and a particularly poor prognosis requiring liver transplantation. The King's College criteria are most commonly used and can be found in Table 20-2. Because of the rapidly progressive course of some cases of acute liver failure, evaluation for liver transplantation should be initiated soon after diagnosis.

KEY POINTS TO REMEMBER

- HAV is spread via the fecal–oral route; in the United States, most outbreaks are associated with contamination of food by food-service workers.
- Most cases of HAV are self-limited, and there is no chronic liver disease associated with HAV.
- In endemic areas such as Asia, the predominant mode of transmission of HBV is vertical. In most Western countries, the major routes of transmission are through unprotected sexual intercourse and injection drug use.
- HBsAg is the hallmark of infection of acute HBV and is detectable 2–6 wks before the onset of symptoms. Persistent elevation beyond 6 mos is indicative of chronic infection.
- Acute HCV often goes unrecognized, as <15% of patients have icteric hepatitis.
- Alcohol can cause a wide spectrum of liver disease, from fatty infiltration to chronic liver disease to alcoholic hepatitis and death. Heavy alcohol intake may induce a severe hepatitis with a 15–50% mortality rate.
- In a patient without complicating factors, 15 g of acetaminophen is necessary to cause clinically significant hepatotoxicity.
- Acetaminophen levels should be drawn ≥ 4 hrs after ingestion and plotted on the Rumack-Matthews nomogram. For patients falling into the potentially toxic range, NAC should be initiated.
- The most common known etiologies of acute liver failure are viral hepatitis and hepatotoxic drugs, although in many cases, a distinct etiology cannot be found.
- The presence of severe coagulopathy, encephalopathy, acidosis, or renal failure carries a very poor prognosis in acute liver failure.

REFERENCES AND SUGGESTED READINGS

Bernal W, Wendon J. Acute liver failure: clinical features and management. *Eur J Gastroenterol Hepatol* 1999;11(9):977–984.

Gill R, Sterling R. Acute liver failure. *J Clin Gastroenterol* 2001;33(3):191–198.

Lee WM. Drug-induced hepatotoxicity. *N Engl J Med* 1995;333:1118–1125.

Lidofsky SD. Fulminant hepatic failure. *Crit Care Clin* 1995;11:415–430.

Maddrey W, Boitnott J, Bedine M. Corticosteroid therapy in alcoholic hepatitis. *Gastroenterology* 1978;75:193.

O'Grady JG, Lake JR, Howdle PD, eds. *Comprehensive Clinical Hepatology*. St. Louis: Mosby, 2000.

Rumack BH, Matthews H. Acetaminophen poisoning. *Pediatrics* 1975;55:871–876.

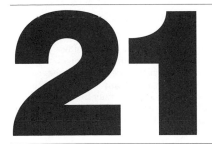

Chronic Liver Disease

Ting-hsu Chen

INTRODUCTION

Chronic liver diseases span a wide variety of conditions, including those of infectious, autoimmune, iatrogenic/drug-induced, and metabolic origin. Successful management of these diseases is particularly challenging to internists and gastroenterologists alike. Early recognition and treatment of these conditions can often prevent or slow progression to more advanced forms of liver disease, including cirrhosis and end-stage liver disease. This chapter focuses on the diagnosis and management of chronic liver diseases. Cirrhosis is discussed in Chap. 22, Cirrhosis.

ALCOHOLIC LIVER DISEASE

Causes

Natural History

Alcoholic liver disease remains one of the most common chronic liver diseases and is second only to hepatitis C (HCV) as an indication for hepatic transplantation. Alcoholic liver disease covers a spectrum of conditions, including fatty liver, alcoholic hepatitis, cirrhosis, and end-stage liver disease. Alcoholic hepatitis and cirrhosis may coexist in the same patient. Early diagnosis and treatment of alcoholic liver disease can result in reversal of all histologic changes in many patients with fatty liver or alcoholic hepatitis. Progression to alcoholic cirrhosis occurs in 8–15% of individuals who consume >50 g alcohol daily (4 oz. of 100-proof whiskey; 15 oz. of wine; four 12-oz. cans of beer) for >10 yrs. A longer duration of alcohol use increases the chance of developing alcoholic hepatitis or cirrhosis.

Concurrent hepatitis B (HBV) or C virus infection or heterozygosity for the hemochromatosis gene (HFE) increases the severity of alcoholic liver disease. The risk of cirrhosis is lower (5%) in the absence of other factors such as chronic viral hepatitis. Genetics account for differences in susceptibility. Women have a lower threshold for development of cirrhosis, even when corrected for body weight.

Presentation

Clinical Presentation

As alcoholic liver disease represents a spectrum, the clinical presentation is variable. Patients with fatty liver often are asymptomatic or have mild right upper quadrant discomfort. Many cases are detected only based on abnormal transaminases. Alcoholic hepatitis typically presents with an acute illness characterized by malaise, abdominal pain, nausea, and vomiting. If severe, ascites or hematemesis (varices) may be present if portal HTN has developed. Portal HTN may be seen in the absence of underlying cirrhosis and often resolves as the alcoholic hepatitis improves. Patients with alcoholic cirrhosis are occasionally asymptomatic but more often have evidence of advanced liver disease, including jaundice, spider angioma, ascites, or encephalopathy.

Management

Diagnostic Evaluation

The diagnosis should be suspected in any patient with a history of alcohol use presenting with the above symptoms. Lab data often support the diagnosis of alcoholic liver disease, but there is no definitive test. Individuals with fatty liver typically have only slightly elevated transaminases, usually with AST greater than ALT. In addition, gamma-glutamyltransferase, transferrin, and mean cell volume may be elevated, but the sensitivity and specificity are limited. U/S often shows abnormal echotexture, consistent with fatty liver. Patients with alcoholic hepatitis have increased transaminases, with AST > ALT but rarely >300. Anemia and leukocytosis are common. Total bilirubin >10 mg/dL and PT >6 secs above control indicate severe disease with up to 50% mortality. Liver biopsy is diagnostic and demonstrates macrovesicular fat, neutrophil infiltration with hepatic necrosis, or Mallory bodies (alcoholic hyaline). Micronodular cirrhosis may be present as well.

Treatment

Abstinence is the cornerstone of treatment, including counseling, dependency programs, and 12-step support groups (e.g., Alcoholics Anonymous). Fatty liver and alcoholic hepatitis are reversible conditions, and many patients with cirrhosis experience improvement in liver function with abstinence from alcohol. Nutritional support is important, as many patients obtain most caloric intake from alcohol and, consequently, have electrolyte and vitamin deficiency. Multivitamin, folic acid, and thiamine supplementation should be provided. As discussed in Chap. 20, Acute Liver Disease, some patients with severe alcoholic hepatitis may benefit from steroids, but this remains controversial. Ultimately, many patients develop end-stage liver disease and should be considered for hepatic transplantation if alcohol intake has been stopped.

CHRONIC VIRAL HEPATITIS

Of the major viruses that cause acute hepatitis, only HBV, HCV, and hepatitis D are associated with chronic hepatitis.

Chronic Hepatitis B

Causes

NATURAL HISTORY. Most adults who contract HBV clear the infection, but approximately 5% develop chronic disease. Immunocompromised adults and young children are at much higher risk for developing chronic HBV. Almost 5% of the world's population is estimated to be infected with chronic HBV. The areas of highest prevalence include Asia and Africa. The risk factors for transmission of the virus include IV drug use, homosexual activity, hemodialysis, and health care workers. Vertical transmission represents the most common mode of infection in endemic areas.

Presentation

CLINICAL PRESENTATION. Unlike patients with acute HBV, many patients with chronic HBV are asymptomatic. Some have nonspecific symptoms, including fatigue, abdominal pain, and arthralgias. If more advanced liver disease has developed, findings consistent with cirrhosis may be present. Other rare complications of chronic HBV include glomerulonephritis, polyarteritis nodosa, and cryoglobulinemia.

Management

DIAGNOSTIC EVALUATION. Routine lab studies usually reveal abnormal transaminases, typically with ALT > AST. Measurement of specific antigens and antibodies forms the basis for determination of HBV infection. See Chap. 20, Acute Liver Disease, for a full description of the markers that are commonly used. The presence of active HBV requires the presence of detectable HBsAg. The other markers allow differentiation into low and active (high) replication conditions (Table 21-1). Liver biopsy allows assessment of degree of inflammation and fibrosis and is typically performed before initiating any antiviral therapy.

TABLE 21-1. MARKERS OF CHRONIC HEPATITIS B (HBV) INFECTION

Low replicative phase
  HBsAg
  IgG antibody against HBV core antigen
  Antibody against HBV e antigen
Active (high) replicative phase
  IgM antibody against HBV core antigen
  HBV e antigen
  High circulating levels of HBV DNA

TREATMENT. Prevention remains the best option for management. Routine immunization of newborns is now performed. High-risk groups, such as IV drug users, dialysis patients, homosexuals, and health care workers, should be offered vaccination. For patients with chronic hepatitis C, it is essential to determine if active replication is present (see Table 21-1). Patients with low viral replication are considered chronic carriers and do not require specific treatment. Individuals with active viral replication are candidates for antiviral therapies. The goals of therapy are seroconversion from HBV e antigen (HBeAg) positivity to anti-HBe positivity, loss of detectable HBV DNA, normalization of ALT, histologic improvement in inflammation and fibrosis, and reduced mortality. The most commonly used agents are interferon (IFN) alpha, lamivudine, and adefovir dipivoxil.

Interferon alpha-2b. IFN is an immunomodulator whose exact effect against hepatitis B is not known. It is given as an SC injection, 5 million U/day or 10 million U three times/wk. Loss of HBeAg and HBV DNA occurs in approximately one-third of patients. Predictors of successful response to therapy are high transaminase levels, low HBV DNA levels, and histology consistent with active hepatitis. There are significant side effects, however, including flu-like illness, leucopenia, thrombocytopenia, thyroid dysfunction, and depression. Patients with a history of major depression should not be treated with IFN because of the risk of severe depression with suicidal ideation.

Lamivudine. A nucleoside analog that inhibits viral reverse transcriptase, lamivudine is effective in decreasing HBV DNA levels at 100 mg/day. It is taken orally and is generally well tolerated without significant side effects. Its long-term efficacy is limited by the development of viral resistance. A mutation in the viral DNA called the *YMDD mutation* develops in more than one-half of all patients treated for 4 yrs with lamivudine, rendering the drug ineffective.

Adefovir Dipivoxil. Adefovir dipivoxil is a newer nucleoside analog that is also effective at decreasing HBV DNA levels at 10 mg PO daily. To date, problems with emergence of viral resistance have not been detected, but more studies are needed.

Chronic Hepatitis C

Causes

NATURAL HISTORY. Since its discovery in 1989, HCV has become a significant public health issue. The virus is estimated to affect 1–2% of the United States population, or >4 million people. It is now known to cause most cases of "non-A, non-B" hepatitis. The main risk factors for transmission include injection drug use, needlestick exposure, snorting cocaine, multiple sexual partners, tattoos, and blood transfusion before 1992. Many individuals have likely been infected for ≥ 20 yrs.

Presentation

CLINICAL PRESENTATION. Most cases of acute HCV infection are asymptomatic or have nonspecific symptoms of malaise, nausea, or vomiting. Only a minority of patients develop an icteric illness. Consequently, most patients do not recall the time of initial infection. However, only 15% of patients clear the virus, and 85% develop chronic infection. Many individuals are diagnosed with chronic HCV based on abnormal liver chemistries followed by confirmatory testing. At the time of diagnosis, many patients have advanced fibrosis or even cirrhosis. The latent period between infection and cirrhosis is variable, but up to 20–30% of patients develop cirrhosis. HCV is currently the most common indication for hepatic transplantation. However, recurrence occurs in all transplanted livers, and the disease is often more aggressive.

Management
DIAGNOSTIC EVALUATION.   The diagnosis should be suspected in any individual with increased transaminases or in high-risk individuals. The anti-HCV antibody is fairly sensitive, but false-positives are common. Consequently, any positive HCV antibody should be confirmed using qualitative and quantitative serum HCV RNA by PCR. Once the diagnosis is confirmed, the genotype should be determined, as it is a strong predictor of response to treatment. Genotype 1 is the most common genotype in the United States, but it has the worst response to treatment. Genotypes 2 and 3 are less common but have a better response rate. All patients being considered for treatment should undergo liver biopsy to determine the degree of inflammation and fibrosis.

TREATMENT.   Therapy should be offered to patients with chronic hepatitis C who have stable disease without evidence of advanced cirrhosis. In addition, individuals with ongoing alcohol or substance abuse, psychiatric illness (especially depression), anemia, or ischemic heart disease should not be given standard therapy due to risk of side effects. Currently, pegylated IFN combined with ribavirin offers the best treatment option. Pegylated IFN alpha-2a or -2b is given as a once-weekly SC injection, and ribavirin is given 800–1200 mg orally each day. If HCV RNA levels are undetectable or have decreased significantly after 12 wks of therapy, treatment is continued for 24 wks (genotype 2 or 3) or 48 wks (genotype 1). A sustained virologic response is defined as normal ALT and undetectable HCV RNA 6 mos after completion of therapy. Predictors of poor response are high levels of HCV RNA, genotype 1, presence of cirrhosis, and ongoing substance abuse (alcohol).

HEREDITARY HEMOCHROMATOSIS

Hereditary hemochromatosis is a common disorder with an incidence of 1 in 200–800. It is an autosomal-recessive disorder that is more common in persons of northern European descent. The autosomal-recessive gene HFE on chromosome 6 encodes a major histocompatibility complex class I–like protein resulting in reduced transferrin receptor affinity for transferrin. The result is chronically increased intestinal iron absorption. 80% of gene mutations are due to a C282Y missense mutation. The average age of presentation is 40–60 yrs, with 20–40 g of excess iron. Men are 10 times more likely to develop significant iron overload due to lack of menses. Complications of iron overload include slate-colored skin, diabetes, cardiomyopathy, arthritis, hypogonadism, or hepatic dysfunction. Patients with cirrhosis due to hemochromatosis are at a significantly increased risk of hepatocellular carcinoma. Almost all patients have elevated serum ferritin levels (men: >300 ng/mL; women: >200 ng/mL) and high transferrin saturation (men: >55%; women: >45%). The diagnosis is confirmed with liver biopsy. The hepatic iron concentration and hepatic iron index are useful measures of hepatic iron stores and are calculated as follows:

$$\text{Hepatic iron concentration } (\mu\text{mol/g}) = \frac{\mu\text{g iron/g dry weight}}{56 \text{ (atomic weight of iron)}}$$

$$\text{Hepatic iron index} = \frac{\text{HIC}}{\text{age (yrs)}}$$

Hepatic iron concentration >4000 μg/g dry weight and hepatic iron index >1.9 are diagnostic. Common genetic mutations (C282Y, H63D) can also be assessed.

Therapy involves phlebotomy of 500 mL whole blood/wk until mild anemia develops and ferritin <50 ng/mL or transferrin saturation <30%. Maintenance phlebotomy of 1–2 units 3–4 times/yr should continue indefinitely. First-degree relatives should be screened if the mutation is detected in the proband or if they have a high serum ferritin or transferrin saturation. Genetic counseling is important, as cirrhosis increases risks for hepatocellular carcinoma despite therapy. Survival of noncirrhotic treated individuals is the same as that of the general population.

AUTOIMMUNE HEPATITIS

Autoimmune hepatitis is a less common cause of chronic liver disease. It commonly affects young women. The most common clinical manifestations are fatigue, jaundice, acne, irregular menses, and hepatomegaly. Diagnosis should be suspected in patients with unexplained elevations of serum transaminases, alkaline phosphatase, and bilirubin. The presence of polyclonal hypergammaglobulinemia is required for diagnosis. Other autoimmune markers may be elevated as well, including ANA, anti–smooth muscle antibody, and anti-LKM1 (liver-kidney-microsomal). Affected individuals may have other manifestations of autoimmune disease, including vasculitis, thyroiditis, or Sjögren's syndrome. Liver biopsy should be performed in suspected cases of autoimmune hepatitis, both to confirm the diagnosis as well as determine the severity of hepatic inflammation. Findings on liver biopsy may include periportal hepatitis, bridging fibrosis, or cirrhosis. Prednisone and azathioprine form the basis for treatment of autoimmune hepatitis. However, even with early diagnosis and treatment, many patients progress to end-stage liver disease and possible hepatic transplantation.

WILSON'S DISEASE

Wilson's disease is a relatively uncommon disease of copper metabolism. It is an autosomal-recessive condition in which mutations of the gene ATP7B on chromosome 13 encoding a copper-transporting adenosine triphosphatase highly expressed in brain and liver result in progressive copper overload. The average age of presentation is 10–15 yrs, with hepatic manifestations typically occurring earlier than neuropsychiatric manifestations. Wilson's disease is rare beyond 40 yrs. Hepatic disease may resemble acute viral hepatitis (sometimes with fulminant hepatic failure), chronic active hepatitis, or postnecrotic cirrhosis. Up to one-third of patients may present with psychiatric manifestations. Other extrahepatic manifestations include Coombs-negative hemolytic anemia in massive copper release, muscular rigidity, dystonic postures, tremor, nephrolithiasis, Fanconi's syndrome, and Kayser-Fleischer corneal rings on slit lamp exam. No test is diagnostic, but complementary results on multiple tests are helpful, including an elevated serum-free copper level (>25 mg/dL), low ceruloplasmin level (<20 mg/dL), elevated 24-hr urinary copper level (>100 μg), or hepatic copper level (>250 μg/g dry weight) on liver biopsy. Management involves zinc salts (150 mg/day PO) to reduce absorption and penicillamine (1–3 g/day PO) or trientine as chelating agents that promote urinary excretion. Treatment should be lifelong, as rapid hepatic and neurologic sequelae may occur with discontinuation of therapy. Neurologic and psychiatric symptoms often improve with treatment, but some residual deficits may persist.

NONALCOHOLIC FATTY LIVER DISEASE

Previously referred to as *nonalcoholic steatohepatitis*, the term **nonalcoholic fatty liver disease (NAFLD)** is now the preferred term. NAFLD represents a spectrum of disorders, including fatty liver, steatohepatitis, and cirrhosis. It commonly affects overweight individuals with diabetes and hyperlipidemia but may occur in persons of normal weight. The prevalence of this disease is increasing as obesity becomes an increasing problem. Most individuals are asymptomatic but may describe mild right upper quadrant discomfort or nausea. As the condition closely mimics alcoholic liver disease, significant alcohol intake must be excluded. Many cases of NAFLD are detected on routine blood testing as elevated transaminases or alkaline phosphatase. Unlike alcoholic liver disease, ALT is usually greater than AST in NAFLD. It currently represents one of the most common causes of abnormal liver chemistries in the United States. U/S may show abnormal liver echotexture, suggestive of fatty infiltration. The diagnosis is based on the finding of moderate to gross macrovesicular fatty degeneration on liver biopsy. Steatohepatitis (sometimes with Mallory bodies) or fibrosis may also be identified of liver biopsy. NAFLD may account for some cases of "cryptogenic" cirrhosis. Other types of liver disease should be excluded, as other entities may present with similar steatosis (HCV, alcoholic liver disease). There is no established therapy, but gradual weight loss, aggressive glycemic control, and antihyperlipidemic agents may be beneficial. Caution must be used with certain lipid-lowering medications (statins), as they may cause increased transaminases and confuse the clinical situation. Gastric bypass or gastroplasty may be considered to treat morbid obesity.

KEY POINTS TO REMEMBER

- Alcoholic liver disease covers a spectrum of conditions, including fatty liver, alcoholic hepatitis, cirrhosis, and end-stage liver disease.
- Fatty liver and alcoholic hepatitis are reversible, and many patient with cirrhosis have significant improvement in liver function after abstaining from alcohol.
- Almost 5% of the world's population is infected with hepatitis B, with vertical transmission being the most common mode of infection in endemic areas.
- Only patients with active viral replication should be offered antiviral treatment in chronic hepatitis B.
- Chronic HCV is the most common indication for hepatic transplantation. It recurs in 100% of transplanted livers.
- Hereditary hemochromatosis is a common disorder caused by a mutation of the HFE gene, resulting in increased iron absorption.
- Wilson's disease is a rare disorder of copper metabolism that may present with liver disease, neuropsychiatric problems, or hemolytic anemia.
- NAFLD represents one of the most common causes of abnormal liver chemistries. It is increasing in prevalence due to the obesity epidemic.

REFERENCES AND SUGGESTED READINGS

Bacon BR. Diagnosis and management of hemochromatosis. *Gastroenterology* 1997; 113:995–999.

Brewer GJ, Yuzbasiyan-Gurkan V. Wilson's disease. *Medicine* 1992;71:139–164.

Desmet VJ, Gerber M, Hoofnagle JH. Classification of chronic hepatitis: diagnosis, grading and staging. *Hepatology* 1994;19:1513–1520.

Diehl AM. Alcoholic liver disease. *Med Clin North Am* 1989;78:815–830.

Flier JS, Underhill LH. Medical disorders of alcoholism. *N Engl J Med* 1995;333: 1058–1065.

Hoofnagle JH, Di Bisceglie AM. Serologic diagnosis of acute and chronic viral hepatitis. *Semin Liver Dis* 1991;11:73–83.

Hoofnagle JH, Di Bisceglie AM. The treatment of chronic viral hepatitis. *N Engl J Med* 1997;336:347–356.

Krawitt EL. Autoimmune hepatitis. *N Engl J Med* 1996;334:897–903.

National Institutes of Health Consensus Development Conference Statement. Management of Hepatitis C 2002. *Gastroenterology* 2002;123:2082–2099.

Sanyal AJ. AGA technical review on nonalcoholic fatty liver disease. *Gastroenterology* 2002;123:1705–1725.

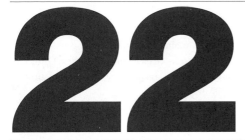

Cirrhosis

Aaron Shiels

INTRODUCTION

Definition

Cirrhosis
The WHO defines cirrhosis as a "diffuse process characterized by fibrosis and conversion of normal liver architecture into structurally abnormal nodules which lack normal lobular organization." Cirrhosis represents the final common end point for many chronic liver diseases and accounts for substantial morbidity and mortality. A multidisciplinary approach involving general internists, gastroenterologists, hepatologists, nurses, dietitians, and social workers is often required to care for these patients due to the complexity of their disease.

Portal Hypertension
The normal portal venous pressure is approximately 5–10 mm Hg, producing a portosystemic gradient of 2–6 mm Hg. Portal HTN is present when the gradient is >12 mm Hg. Cirrhosis is the most common cause of portal HTN in the United States, but there are many other causes that must be excluded. The causes of portal HTN can be divided into prehepatic, intrahepatic, and posthepatic causes. Prehepatic causes include portal vein and splenic vein thrombosis. Intrahepatic causes are viral hepatitis, primary biliary cirrhosis, cirrhosis, alcoholic hepatitis, venoocclusive disease, and schistosomiasis (most common etiology worldwide). Common posthepatic causes are Budd-Chiari syndrome, vascular invasion, and constrictive pericarditis.

CAUSES

Pathophysiology

Liver damage occurs through a variety of mechanisms and may occur at the level of the hepatocyte, bile duct, artery, sinusoid, vein, or lymphatics. The liver has a tremendous regenerative capacity, even to the point of allowing half of the liver to regenerate after partial hepatectomy in living liver donors. However, when diffuse and prolonged damage occurs, the liver ultimately develops regenerative nodules and fibrosis leading to cirrhosis. Regardless of the type of injury, the common end point is irreversible damage to the liver with micronodular or macronodular cirrhosis. The classic findings on liver biopsy include regenerating nodules, fibrosis, and abnormal hepatic architecture. The abnormal architecture causes disruption of the normal blood flow through the liver, resulting in portal HTN and portosystemic shunting. This accounts for many of the complications of cirrhosis, including esophageal varices, ascites, splenomegaly, and portosystemic encephalopathy (PSE). In addition, the remaining hepatocytes do not function normally, resulting in synthetic dysfunction with hypoalbuminemia and coagulopathy. Aside from the more common complications, cirrhosis can affect many organ systems (Table 22-1).

TABLE 22-1. MANIFESTATIONS OF CIRRHOSIS

Constitutional	Fatigue, weight loss, anorexia, malaise, muscle wasting
GI	Esophageal varices, portal hypertensive gastropathy, ascites, GI bleed
Pulmonary	Hypoxia, hepatopulmonary syndrome, respiratory alkalosis, pleural effusion, portopulmonary HTN
Cardiovascular	Hypotension, hyperdynamic circulation
Renal	Hepatorenal syndrome, sodium retention with edema, hyponatremia
Endocrine	Decreased libido, impotence, testicular atrophy, dysmenorrhea, gynecomastia
Neurologic	Encephalopathy, asterixis, hyperreflexia
Dermatologic	Spider angioma, palmar erythema, jaundice, Dupuytren's contracture
Hematologic	Splenomegaly, thrombocytopenia, anemia, leukopenia, coagulopathy

PRESENTATION

Clinical Presentation

Cirrhosis

Patients may present with a broad range of symptoms, including any combination of the manifestations listed in Table 22-1. Some patients present for evaluation of other problems and are incidentally found to have physical findings or lab abnormalities suggestive of cirrhosis. The initial evaluation should include a thorough history and physical exam aimed at determining whether the patient has cirrhosis and identifying possible etiologies. A multitude of diseases can lead to cirrhosis, but in the United States, most cases are due to alcoholic liver disease or chronic viral hepatitis. Table 22-2 lists the

TABLE 22-2. CAUSES OF CIRRHOSIS AND CLUES TO DIAGNOSIS

Alcoholic liver disease	History of prolonged alcohol intake, increased AST to ALT ratio
Chronic viral hepatitis	Hepatitis B and C serologies
Primary biliary cirrhosis	Hypercholesterolemia, antimitochondrial antibody
Primary sclerosing cholangitis	History of ulcerative colitis, increased alkaline phosphatase
Hemochromatosis	Iron studies, HFE gene mutations
Alpha$_1$-antitrypsin deficiency	Positive family history, phenotype testing (PiZZ phenotype)
Wilson's disease	Kaiser-Fleisher rings, low serum ceruloplasmin, high urinary copper
Autoimmune hepatitis	ANA, increased serum quantitative Igs
Cryptogenic cirrhosis	Absence of other causes
Nonalcoholic fatty liver disease	Diabetes mellitus, obesity, hyperlipidemia
Jejunoileal bypass	History of obesity surgery
Drugs	History of methotrexate, amiodarone
Budd-Chiari syndrome	Hypercoagulable state, nephrotic syndrome, paroxysmal nocturnal hemoglobinuria
Venoocclusive disease	Stem-cell transplant

most common causes of cirrhosis and specific clues to diagnosis. Specifically, patients should be asked about duration and quantity of alcohol intake, risk factors for viral hepatitis, family history of liver disease, and prescription and over-the-counter drug use. If cirrhosis is suspected, the workup should also focus on identifying complications. The physical exam is often very helpful and often demonstrates muscle wasting, gynecomastia, spider angioma, asterixis, and jaundice, especially in patients with advanced cirrhosis. Initial labs should include transaminases, alkaline phosphatase, bilirubin, electrolytes, creatinine, protime and albumin. A specific etiology may be found with viral hepatitis serologies, iron studies, ceruloplasmin, serum quantitative Igs, ANAs, antimitochondrial antibodies, or $alpha_1$-antitrypsin phenotype studies. Because cirrhosis of any cause increases risk for hepatocellular carcinoma, all patients should have an AFP level and imaging study. The imaging studies are also useful for assessing the size of the liver and biliary tree. In many patients, the diagnosis of cirrhosis can be made with certainty based on history, exam, and basic lab and imaging studies. A liver biopsy may provide information regarding etiology.

Portal Hypertension

Most cases of portal HTN can be diagnosed on the basis of clinical features. Patients present with any of the manifestations of portal HTN, including upper GI bleeding from varices or portal hypertensive gastropathy, ascites, splenomegaly with hypersplenism, or encephalopathy. All patients with suspected portal HTN should undergo an evaluation to determine etiology. This should include an U/S to evaluate the liver parenchyma and document patency of the portal and hepatic veins. An attempt should be made to identify all possible complications of portal HTN. Only rarely do patients require direct measurement of the portosystemic pressure gradient. If necessary, this can be done by transjugular cannulation of the hepatic veins.

MANAGEMENT

Treatment

Cirrhosis is an irreversible condition, so treatment is largely supportive and aimed at treating or preventing the numerous complications. In some cases, specific treatments may improve overall liver function. Patients with alcoholic liver disease must quit drinking. Many presumed cirrhotics have substantial improvement after abstaining from alcohol. Specific antiviral therapy may be of some benefit in selected patients with chronic hepatitis B or C. All patients should receive surveillance AFP and imaging study every 6–12 mos. Suspicious lesions should then undergo CT- or U/S-guided liver biopsy to rule out hepatocellular carcinoma. Vaccinations against hepatitis A and B should be given. The specific complications are discussed in the following sections. Ultimately, many patients progress to end-stage liver disease and may be referred for transplantation. Liver failure due to cirrhosis is often graded according to the Child-Turcotte-Pugh (CTP) scoring system (Table 22-3). Patients with Child's class C liver disease (CTP score ≥ 10) have a substantial operative mortality.

Complications

Most of the complications of cirrhosis are related to portal HTN. Therefore, the management of cirrhosis and portal HTN is largely directed toward preventing and treating the complications.

Esophageal Varices

Patients with portal HTN often develop portosystemic collaterals in the retroperitoneum, internal hemorrhoids, and falciform ligament (caput medusae). However, the most clinically significant portosystemic collaterals occur at the esophagogastric junction, resulting in dilated esophageal veins, or varices. Approximately 70% of cirrhotics develop esophageal varices, and 30% of these patients eventually bleed. Patients who have a first variceal bleed are at a significant risk for recurrent bleeding. Increased

TABLE 22-3. CHILD-TURCOTTE-PUGH SCORING SYSTEM

Criteria	1	2	3
Ascites	None	Slight	Moderate-severe
Encephalopathy	None	Mild	Moderate-severe
Bilirubin (mg/dL)	<2	2–3	>3
Albumin (g/dL)	>3.5	2.8–3.5	<2.8
Protime (secs above normal protime)	1–3	4–6	>6

Note: Child's class determined by adding scores from each of the five criteria together: class A, 5–6 points; class B, 7–9 points; class C, 10–15 points.

risk of bleeding occurs with large varices, endoscopic red color signs, advanced Child's class, and active alcohol use. Management of varices can be divided into acute bleeding and long-term treatment.

ACUTE VARICEAL BLEEDING. As with all GI bleeding, the immediate focus should be on resuscitation of the patient. In patients with suspected variceal bleeding, there are special points that deserve emphasis. Due to the presence of liver disease, coagulopathy with elevated protime and thrombocytopenia are common and should be corrected with vitamin K, FFP, or platelets as needed. Care must be used not to overtransfuse, as increased blood volume has the theoretic risk of increasing bleeding risk. Octreotide (Sandostatin) (50–100 μg IV bolus, 25–50 μg/hr) is a somatostatin analog that decreases splanchnic pressure and should be started if variceal bleeding is suspected. It is fairly effective at decreasing the bleeding risk and is much safer than vasopressin and nitroglycerin. If sepsis or **spontaneous bacterial peritonitis (SBP)** is suspected, then antibiotics may be required after appropriate blood and fluid cultures have been obtained. Once patients have been adequately resuscitated and coagulopathy corrected, upper endoscopy should be performed. This allows both diagnostic and therapeutic capabilities. Many patients require intubation for airway protection during the procedure. Endoscopic variceal ligation (banding) has largely replaced sclerotherapy in the management of acute variceal bleeding. If endoscopy is not immediately available or if the bleeding cannot be stopped with medical and endoscopic management, then balloon tamponade may provide temporary control. However, this has a high risk of complications, including aspiration and asphyxiation, and must be used cautiously. For patients refractory to these measures, emergent transhepatic portosystemic shunting (TIPS) can be performed to decompress the varices.

LONG-TERM TREATMENT. Primary prophylaxis can help to prevent an initial bleeding episode, especially in patients with large varices. This involves nonselective beta blockers (nadolol, propranolol), which have been shown to decrease portal pressure and the size of the varices. Prophylactic endoscopic ligation provides another option for decreasing the risk of a first bleed. Because of the high rate of recurrent bleeding, secondary prophylaxis is important after the first bleeding episode. Beta blockers should be used in patients with Child's class A or B cirrhosis who are compliant with no absolute contraindications to beta blockers. A long-acting nitrate, such as isosorbide mononitrate, can also be added. Repeat endoscopic ligation until the varices have been obliterated is also useful. It is not clear whether medical management or endoscopic therapy (or both) provides the lowest risk of bleeding. Patients who have recurrent bleeding should be considered as candidates for TIPS or a surgical shunt.

Ascites and Spontaneous Bacterial Peritonitis

Ascites is the abnormal accumulation of fluid within the peritoneal cavity. There are numerous causes of ascites, but cirrhosis with portal HTN is the most common etiology. The diagnosis and management of ascites is detailed in Chap. 12, Ascites. SBP is a complication that deserves special mention. SBP commonly develops in cirrhotic patients with ascites. Increased risk for SBP is seen with ascitic total protein <1 mg/ dL, variceal hemorrhage, or prior episodes of SBP. Presentation may be subtle with generalized abdominal pain, fever, chills, jaundice, or worsening encephalopathy. All patients with suspected SBP should undergo diagnostic paracentesis with inoculation of blood culture bottles at the bedside, as this greatly increases the sensitivity of cultures. An ascitic fluid total WBC >500 cells/μL or neutrophil count >250 cells/μL is required for the diagnosis of SBP. Gram-negative bacilli and streptococci account for the majority of cases of SBP. Empiric antibiotics (cefotaxime or ceftriaxone) should be started after fluid and blood are sent for culture. Repeat paracentesis is required at day 5 if the patient does not improve clinically or if secondary peritonitis is suspected. Antibiotics are usually continued for 10–14 days, but studies suggest 5 days may be adequate. One study also demonstrated decreased mortality in patients treated with IV albumin. The role of prophylactic antibiotics, such as fluoroquinolones, remains controversial but should be considered for the high-risk groups mentioned above.

Encephalopathy

Hepatic encephalopathy or PSE presents one of the most challenging and disabling aspects of cirrhosis and portal HTN. The exact mechanism remains controversial, but it is likely related to impaired hepatic detoxification of neurotoxins through a combination of decreased hepatocyte function and portosystemic shunting. The encephalopathy associated with chronic liver disease tends to be more insidious, with recurrent episodes that are usually reversible. This is somewhat different from the fulminant encephalopathy seen in patients with acute liver failure. PSE symptoms range from mild sleep disturbances or personality changes to more severe forms with lethargy or coma. PSE is generally graded from I to IV, as in Table 22-4. Most patients have other manifestations of chronic liver disease, and the diagnosis can usually be made on clinical grounds with altered mental status, asterixis, and hypo- or hyperreflexia. Other causes of encephalopathy should be excluded. Ammonia levels have very poor specificity and should not be used to diagnose PSE or monitor treatment response. Management should be directed at identifying and treating possible precipitating factors, as in Table 22-5. Empiric treatment with lactulose should be started in all patients with suspected PSE. The dose of lactulose should be titrated to produce 3–4 loose stools/ day. Patients with refractory PSE present difficult management issues. Attempts should be made to identify precipitants that may have been missed. Lactulose may be given by NG tube or retention enemas if patients cannot drink enough lactulose to produce loose stools.

Coagulopathy

Several factors contribute to the increased bleeding risk seen in patients with cirrhosis and portal HTN. The liver synthesizes most of the clotting factors, and decreased hepatocyte function results in abnormally low levels of these factors. Intrahepatic cholestasis is commonly seen in cirrhosis and may cause vitamin K deficiency. Decreased levels of clotting factors and vitamin K deficiency contribute to abnormal clotting cascade, usually measured as prolonged protime. Thrombocytopenia is present in at least one-third of cirrhotics and is primarily due to hypersplenism, with sequestration of platelets within the enlarged spleen. In addition, the remaining platelets do not function nor-

TABLE 22-4. GRADES OF ENCEPHALOPATHY

Grade	Characteristics
I	Sleep reversal pattern, mild confusion, irritability, tremor
II	Lethargy, disorientation, inappropriate behavior, asterixis
III	Somnolence, severe confusion, aggressive behavior, asterixis
IV	Comatose

TABLE 22-5.   COMMON PRECIPITANTS OF ENCEPHALOPATHY

GI bleeding	Post–transhepatic portosystemic shunting
Constipation	Hepatocellular carcinoma
Infection (including SBP)	Worsening hepatic function
Prerenal azotemia	Benzodiazepines
Hypokalemia	Narcotics
Alkalosis	Diuretic use

SBP, spontaneous bacterial peritonitis.

mally. Finally, many patients may have a variant of consumptive coagulopathy similar to disseminated intravascular coagulation. All of these factors contribute to an increased risk of epistaxis, gingival bleeding, ecchymoses, and GI bleeding. Correction of these abnormalities plays a critical role in management of cirrhotics with significant hemorrhage, especially GI bleeding. In addition, special attention must be given to optimizing coagulation parameters before elective or emergent procedures. This is best accomplished with a combination of vitamin K, FFP, and platelets. Vitamin K may be ineffective in patients with severely impaired synthetic function.

Hepatorenal Syndrome
Patients with advanced cirrhosis and portal HTN may present with a progressive renal failure termed **hepatorenal syndrome (HRS).** This is a condition whose cause is unknown. There is a chronic form seen in advanced cirrhotics and an acute form seen in severe alcoholic hepatitis or fulminant hepatic failure. The chronic form typically presents as worsening azotemia associated with diuretic-resistant edema. It is essential to exclude other potentially treatable causes of renal failure, such as prerenal azotemia, acute tubular necrosis, nephrotoxins, and glomerulopathies. Most patients have oliguric renal failure with low urine sodium and bland urinary sediment. Differentiation between HRS and prerenal azotemia is often difficult, and all patients should receive a trial of volume expansion. If the diagnosis remains unclear, then central venous pressure monitoring may be required. Treatment is aimed at correction of potentially reversible factors, adequate volume resuscitation, and avoidance of additional nephrotoxic agents. Many patients require liver transplantation. Renal function generally returns to normal after transplantation. HRS carries a very poor prognosis, with a median survival of only 10–14 days.

KEY POINTS TO REMEMBER

- The abnormal architecture found in cirrhosis causes disruption of the normal blood flow through the liver, resulting in portal HTN and portosystemic shunting.
- Cirrhosis of any cause increases risk for hepatocellular carcinoma, and all patients should have an AFP level and imaging study (U/S, CT, or MRI) every 6–12 mos.
- Cirrhosis is an irreversible condition, so treatment is largely supportive and aimed at treating or preventing the numerous complications.
- Approximately 70% of cirrhotics develop esophageal varices, and 30% of these patients eventually bleed. The mortality for each episode of bleeding approaches 50%.
- Octreotide is a somatostatin analog that decreases splanchnic pressure and should be started if variceal bleeding is suspected.
- Medical therapy with beta blockers and nitrates and endoscopic therapy with variceal ligation are useful for primary and secondary prophylaxis of esophageal variceal bleeding.
- An ascitic fluid total WBC >500 cells/μL or neutrophil count >250 cells/μL is required for the diagnosis of SBP.
- Empiric treatment with lactulose should be started in all patients with suspected PSE. The dose of lactulose should be titrated to produce 3–4 loose stools/day.

- Thrombocytopenia is present in at least one-third of cirrhotics and is primarily due to hypersplenism with sequestration of platelets within the enlarged spleen.
- HRS carries a very poor prognosis, with a median survival of only 10–14 days.

REFERENCES AND SUGGESTED READINGS

Anthony PP, Ishak NG, Nayak NC, et al. The morphology of cirrhosis: recommendations on definition, nomenclature, and classification by a working group sponsored by the World Health Organization. *J Clin Pathol* 1978;31:395–414.

Arroyo V, Gines P, Gerbes AL. Definition and diagnostic criteria of refractory ascites and hepatorenal syndrome in cirrhosis. *Hepatology* 1996;23:164–176.

Cordoba J, Blei AT. Treatment of hepatic encephalopathy. *Am J Gastroenterol* 1997; 92:1429–1439.

D'Amico G, Pagliaro L, Bosch J. The treatment of portal hypertension: a meta-analytic review. *Hepatology* 1995;22:332–351.

Grace ND. Management of portal hypertension. *Gastroenterologist* 1993;1:39–58.

Guarner C, Runyon BA. Spontaneous bacterial peritonitis: pathogenesis, diagnosis. *Gastroenterologist* 1995;3:311–328.

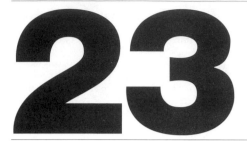

Pancreatic Disorders

Sandeep K. Tripathy

INTRODUCTION

The pancreas is a mixed endocrine and exocrine gland consisting of lobular subunits composed of acini. The exocrine pancreas consists of acinar, centroacinar, and ductal cells. The acinar cells secrete approximately 20 digestive enzymes (in zymogen granules) into the central ductule of the acinus, which then connects with the intralobular ducts to form the interlobular ducts; these ducts, in turn, form the main pancreatic duct. This then empties into the duodenum through the ampulla of Vater. Diseases of the pancreas are generally more difficult to manage medically or surgically than those of other abdominal viscera. The pancreas lies in the retroperitoneal space of the upper abdomen. The central position of the pancreas provides for lymphatic drainage along several major routes (the splenic, hepatic, and superior mesenteric nodal systems as well as the aortocaval and other posterior abdominal wall lymphatic vessels). The association with vital major vessels of the epigastrium also makes diseases of the pancreas difficult to treat. When a tumor spreads a short distance to involve the superior mesenteric vein, the portal vein, or the celiac axis, it usually becomes incurable. If the gland is removed, the need to excise the vessels and lymph nodes associated with it often makes it necessary to remove the duodenum, gallbladder, distal bile duct, spleen, upper jejunum, and part of the stomach. Finally, the vascular nature of the pancreas and the adjacent organs makes hemorrhage the most common periop complication of pancreatic resection.

ACUTE PANCREATITIS

Causes

Pathophysiology

The incidence of acute pancreatitis ranges from 1–5/10,000 per year. Two histologic forms of acute pancreatitis are recognized: acute interstitial and acute hemorrhagic. In interstitial pancreatitis, the gland is edematous, but its gross architecture is preserved, and hemorrhage is absent. In the acute hemorrhagic form, marked tissue necrosis and hemorrhage are apparent. Surrounding areas of fat necrosis are also prominent. Large hematomas are often seen in the retroperitoneal space. Vascular inflammation and thrombosis are common. Mortality is more likely with the hemorrhagic form.

Processes that contribute to the initiation of pancreatitis include pancreatic duct obstruction, pancreatic ischemia, and the premature activation of zymogens within the pancreatic acinar cells. Acute pancreatitis has been considered an autodigestive process that occurs when the proteolytic enzymes are activated in the pancreas rather than in the intestinal lumen. The active enzymes then digest membranes within the pancreas, leading to edema, vascular damage, cellular injury, and death. This, in turn, leads to the further release of inflammatory cytokines (tumor necrosis factor, interleukin-1, platelet-activating factor), which causes the recruitment of inflammatory cells and increases vascular permeability. In this manner, a cascade of events leads to the development of acute necrotizing pancreatitis. Most cases of mild acute pancreatitis are self-limited, with a mortality of 1%. Patients with severe, necrotizing pancreatitis often have a very complicated hospital course, with a mortality up to 30%.

Differential Diagnosis
GALLSTONES. Gallstone disease and excessive alcohol use combined account for 70–80% of cases of acute pancreatitis in industrialized countries. Although gallstones are etiologically linked to pancreatitis, this condition develops in only a small percentage of patients with gallstones.

ALCOHOL. A single binge use of alcohol rarely, if ever, causes pancreatitis. Alcohol-induced pancreatitis occurs in persons with long-standing alcohol use. Because only approximately 5% of chronic heavy alcohol users develop pancreatitis, other hereditary or environmental risk factors must play a role.

DRUGS. Commonly implicated drugs include azathioprine, 6-mercaptopurine, L-asparaginase, pentamidine, didanosine, valproic acid, furosemide, sulfonamides, tetracyclines, estrogens, metronidazole, and erythromycin.

INFECTION. The most common viral infections that involve the pancreas are mumps and Coxsackie B virus. Viral hepatitis, especially hepatitis B, has been associated with pancreatitis. Clinical pancreatitis occurs in <10% of all patients with AIDS and even fewer of those not receiving toxic medications (hyperamylasemia has been reported in up to 40% of AIDS patients). Bacteria associated with acute pancreatitis include *Salmonella*, *Shigella*, *Campylobacter*, hemorrhagic *Escherichia coli*, *Legionella*, *Leptospira*, and even *Brucella* species. Pancreatitis associated with these infections is most likely secondary to released toxins.

TRAUMA. Acute pancreatitis can be seen after blunt or penetrating abdominal trauma. Iatrogenic causes include endoscopic retrograde cholangiopancreatography (ERCP), pancreaticobiliary surgery, or cardiopulmonary bypass.

HYPERLIPIDEMIA. The breakdown products of triglycerides are responsible for inducing pancreatitis. When lipase in the pancreatic capillary bed acts on the high levels of triglycerides in the serum, toxic free fatty acids are generated. Although triglyceride levels >2000–3000 mg/dL usually are required for development of pancreatitis, it can occur when serum levels are only 500 mg/dL. In general, a level of >1000 mg/dL suggests hyperlipidemia as a cause of the pancreatitis.

IDIOPATHIC. As many as 30% of cases of acute pancreatitis have no identifiable etiology.

Presentation

History and Physical Exam
The hallmark of acute pancreatitis is abdominal pain that is typically located in the epigastrium and periumbilical area and radiates to the back. The pain is frequently more intense when the patient is supine and may be relieved if the patient leans forward or brings both knees to the chest. The pain is usually made worse by the ingestion of food and alcohol. Nausea, emesis, and abdominal distention are also frequently reported. Hematemesis, melena, and diarrhea are infrequent. On physical exam, abdominal tenderness ranges from mild epigastric tenderness to rigidity with rebound tenderness depending on the severity of the presentation. Scleral icterus may be seen because of biliary obstruction or accompanying liver disease. Faint bluish discoloration around the umbilicus (Cullen's sign) or flank (Turner's sign) may rarely be seen in acute hemorrhagic pancreatitis but can also be seen in patients with a ruptured abdominal aortic aneurysm.

Management

Diagnostic Evaluation
BLOOD TESTS. Amylase and lipase are enzymes that are released from the pancreas during acute pancreatitis. Lipase has slightly superior sensitivity and specificity than amylase. Plasma levels of both enzymes peak at 24 hrs of symptoms, but amylase has a shorter half-life.

TABLE 23-1. RANSON'S CRITERIA

On admission	Within 48 hrs
Age >55 yrs	Hct decrease by 10%
WBC >16,000/mm^3	Urea nitrogen increase by >5 mg/dL
Lactate dehydrogenase >350 IU/L	Serum calcium <8 mg/dL
Glucose >200 mg/dL	Arterial PO_2 <60 mm Hg
AST >250 IU/L	Base deficit >4 mEq/L
	Estimated fluid sequestration >6 L

ABDOMINAL IMAGING. U/S has low sensitivity for diagnosing pancreatitis, but it is very useful in determining whether gallstone disease is present as a potential cause (demonstration of stone in the gallbladder or common bile duct dilatation). The CT scan may be normal in up to 30% of patients with mild pancreatitis, but it is almost always abnormal in patients with moderate or severe disease. Diagnostic CT should be performed using a **pancreatic protocol,** which involves thin slices through the pancreas with several contrast phases. Important findings include pancreatic swelling, peripancreatic infiltrates, peripancreatic fluid collections, and areas of nonenhancement of the pancreas.

PREDICTORS OF SEVERITY. Several approaches have been used to differentiate those patients that have a mild course from those that have a more serious illness. This includes Ranson's criteria (Table 23-1), modified Glasgow criteria, and Acute Physiologic and Chronic Health Evaluation (APACHE) II score. When compared at 48 hrs after admission, the three systems are similar. The APACHE II score, however, can be calculated anytime during admission to monitor improvement. None of these methods is better than close observation and clinical judgment.

Treatment

MILD ACUTE PANCREATITIS. Treatment is supportive with bed rest, no oral intake, IV hydration, electrolyte replacement, and analgesia (meperidine or morphine). NG suction may be useful to alleviate the symptoms of nausea, emesis, and abdominal distention. The patient can be cautiously fed once the abdominal pain resolves and the amylase and lipase levels start to return to normal.

SEVERE ACUTE PANCREATITIS. Treatment is also primarily supportive, as for mild disease, except patients with severe acute pancreatitis usually require vigorous resuscitation with fluids. Patients may require intensive care. Large doses of narcotics may be required for pain management. Other treatment modalities are discussed below.

Antibiotics. Prophylactic antibiotics are recommended in cases of necrotizing pancreatitis or associated cholangitis. Antibiotics are not recommended for mild pancreatitis. Appropriate antibiotics should be active against a wide variety of organisms—in particular, gram-negative organisms. The most commonly used regimens include imipenem or a combination of a quinolone and metronidazole.

Endoscopic Retrograde Cholangiopancreatography. ERCP should be performed for possible sphincterotomy and stone extraction in patients with presumed gallstone pancreatitis or findings suggestive of cholangitis (right upper quadrant abdominal pain and tenderness, fever >39°C, leukocyte count >20,000). The timing should be as early as safely possible and no later than 72 hrs after admission.

Enteral Nutrition. After approximately 3–4 days, if the patient does not appear to be able to take food orally, attempts should be made to feed the patient enterally through the jejunum (beyond the ligament of Treitz). This can be accomplished by placement of a nasojejunal feeding tube.

Surgical Débridement. Patients may develop septic complications resulting from infected pancreatic necrosis or abscess formation. They present at least 1 wk into the course with worsening pain, fever, and an elevated WBC. CT scan should be performed with aspiration of any low-density areas or fluid collections. The aspirate should be sent for culture and Gram's stain. If organisms or polymorphonuclear neutrophils are seen, the patient should undergo surgical débridement. The viscous and loculated nature of the fluid tends to make catheter or endoscopic drainage inadequate. Pseudocysts may also develop in 15% of patients. Previously, any pseudocyst >6 cm that persisted for 6 wks was managed with a drainage procedure. However, it now seems appropriate to manage pseudocysts that are not enlarging conservatively with serial CT scans.

CHRONIC PANCREATITIS

Causes

Pathophysiology
Chronic pancreatitis is an inflammatory disease of the pancreas that is characterized by irreversible damage of the pancreatic architecture. This includes irregular fibrosis, acinar cell loss, islet cell loss, and inflammatory cell infiltrates. The incidence of chronic pancreatitis is approximately 4/100,000 per year. The prevalence is approximately 13/100,000. Alcohol in Western societies (70–80%) and malnutrition worldwide are the major etiologies of chronic pancreatitis. In general, prolonged alcohol intake is required to produce symptomatic chronic pancreatitis (6–12 yrs). See Table 23-2 for the TIGAR-O classification system for etiologic risk factors for chronic pancreatitis.

Presentation

Clinical Presentation
ABDOMINAL PAIN. The presenting symptom of most patients with chronic pancreatitis is abdominal pain. The pain is usually epigastric, dull, and constant. The pain may radiate directly to the back. Pain attacks can occur for several days' duration with intervening pain-free intervals, or they may be nearly constant. The aggravation of pain by eating is characteristic of chronic pancreatitis. Although eating may aggravate the pain in other abdominal conditions (e.g., irritable bowel syndrome), there is usually a much greater interval between the meal and the discomfort than is the case with pancreatic disease. Pain in chronic pancreatitis may continue, diminish, or disappear completely. Chronic pancreatitis is painless in approximately 15% of patients. Idiopathic pancreatitis is more likely to be painless than is the alcoholic variety.

TABLE 23-2. TIGAR-O CLASSIFICATION SYSTEM OF CHRONIC PANCREATITIS

Toxic-metabolic	Alcohol, tobacco, hypercalcemia, hyperlipidemia, chronic renal failure, medications (phenacetin abuse)
Idiopathic	Early onset, late onset, tropical
Genetic	Cationic trypsinogen, cystic fibrosis transmembrane conductance regulator mutations
Autoimmune	Sjögren's syndrome, inflammatory bowel disease, primary biliary cirrhosis
Recurrent and severe acute pancreatitis	Postnecrotic, recurrent acute pancreatitis, vascular disease, postirradiation
Obstructive	Pancreas divisum, duct obstruction (tumor), posttraumatic pancreatic duct scars, preampullary duodenal wall cysts

WEIGHT LOSS. Nausea, vomiting, anorexia, and weight loss are common in chronic pancreatitis. Weight loss is usually secondary to decreased caloric intake because of fear of worsening abdominal pain. Malabsorption or uncontrolled diabetes also may play a role in weight loss.

MALABSORPTION. When exocrine secretion of pancreatic enzymes is reduced to <10%, diarrhea, steatorrhea, and azotorrhea can occur. These symptoms tend to occur relatively late in the course of chronic pancreatitis. Fecal weight tends to be less in pancreatic malabsorption than in other conditions with comparable steatorrhea. Patients may pass bulky, formed stool as opposed to the frank watery diarrhea observed in other conditions.

PANCREATIC DIABETES. Clinically evident diabetes occurs relatively late in the disease and occurs in 60% of patients with chronic pancreatitis. Diabetic ketoacidosis and diabetic nephropathy are relatively uncommon in this form of diabetes.

OTHER CLINICAL FEATURES. Less common manifestations of chronic pancreatitis include jaundice (extrinsic bile duct obstruction), ascites, pleural effusion, painful subcutaneous nodules (pancreatic panniculitis), and polyarthritis of the small joints of the hands.

The **physical exam** usually is of limited assistance in the diagnosis of chronic pancreatitis because the intensity of the patient's complaint tends to be out of proportion to the physical signs. Epigastric tenderness may be present during the painful episodes as well as during periods of remission. Complications of chronic pancreatitis (ascites or pleural effusions) may be detected on physical exam.

Management

Diagnostic Evaluation

The diagnosis of chronic pancreatitis often can be made on the basis of history and relatively simple radiographic tests.

Routine blood studies usually are not helpful in making the diagnosis of chronic pancreatitis. Leukocytosis may be observed during acute exacerbations. Anemia and fat-soluble vitamin deficiency states (hypocalcemia, hypoprothrombinemia) are seldom seen in association with the steatorrhea of chronic pancreatitis. Varying degrees of cholestasis can be seen secondary to compression of the common duct by a fibrotic process in the pancreas. This can cause an elevation in serum alkaline phosphatase. Clinical jaundice results from more severe compression.

AMYLASE AND LIPASE. In contrast to attacks of acute pancreatitis, in which the serum level of pancreatic enzymes is almost always elevated, serum enzyme levels may be elevated, normal, or low in chronic pancreatitis.

PLASMA CONCENTRATION OF PANCREATIC POLYPEPTIDE. Pancreatic polypeptide is induced by protein ingestion and cholecystokinin (CCK) administration. A subnormal rise in plasma pancreatic polypeptide after stimulation with a protein-rich meal or secretin infusion is an indicator of chronic pancreatitis.

INDIRECT TESTS OF PANCREATIC EXOCRINE SECRETION. Most of the indirect tests of pancreatic exocrine secretion measure the absorption of some compound that first requires digestion by pancreatic enzymes. Because clinically detectable malabsorption of nutrients does not occur until pancreatic enzyme secretion has diminished to <10% of normal, tests of pancreatic function are unable to detect early chronic pancreatitis.

- The bentiromide test involves ingestion of N-benzoyl-L-tyrosyl-p-aminobenzoic acid (NBT-PABA), a tripeptide that is digested by chymotrypsin with the release of paraaminobenzoic acid (PABA). Free PABA is absorbed in the small bowel and excreted by the kidney. The quantity excreted in urine is used as a measure of pancreatic exocrine function.
- Approximately 40% of patients with chronic pancreatitis have cobalamin (vitamin B_{12}) malabsorption, which is corrected with administration of oral pancreatic enzymes.
- The diagnosis of pancreatic insufficiency by way of measurements of fecal chymotrypsin is rapid and simple. The measurement of total fecal chymotrypsin output in

timed fecal collections appears to offer little advantage over the much simpler measurement of chymotrypsin concentration in a random fecal sample.

Imaging Studies

ABDOMINAL PLAIN FILMS. The evaluation should begin with a plain film of the abdomen. The demonstration of diffuse, speckled calcification of the pancreas on a plain film of the abdomen is diagnostic of chronic pancreatitis, and no further testing is required.

ULTRASOUND. Findings on U/S that correlate with marked pancreatic changes on ERCP include dilation of the main pancreatic duct to >4 mm, large (>1 cm) cavities, and calcifications. When a satisfactory U/S exam is obtained, the reported sensitivity of this test for chronic pancreatitis is approximately 70%, and the specificity is 90%. The finding of chronic pancreatitis on U/S usually requires no additional confirmatory testing.

CT SCAN. CT is more sensitive than U/S for the diagnosis of chronic pancreatitis. CT is more expensive than U/S and involves exposure to ionizing radiation. Therefore, in the workup for chronic pancreatitis, CT usually should be limited to patients who have negative or unsatisfactory U/S exams. The most common diagnostic findings of chronic pancreatitis on CT include duct dilation, calcifications, and cystic lesions. Less common diagnostic findings include enlargement or atrophy of the pancreas and heterogeneous density of the parenchyma.

ENDOSCOPIC RETROGRADE CHOLANGIOPANCREATOGRAPHY. ERCP is commonly considered to be the most sensitive and specific test available for the diagnosis of chronic pancreatitis, and this technique has become the gold standard against which all other tests are evaluated. In mild pancreatitis, the changes are limited to the branches and fine ducts, which show dilation and irregularity. Moderate pancreatitis is characterized by the additional finding of dilation, tortuosity, and stenosis of the main pancreatic duct. Advanced pancreatitis has the additional findings of cyst formation and contraction of the pancreas. In general, there is a good correlation between the changes observed on ERCP and measurements of pancreatic secretory capacity. Because ERCP is an expensive procedure and has a low, but not insignificant, rate of associated complications, this test ordinarily should be reserved for the rare patient with chronic pancreatitis in whom the diagnosis cannot be clearly established by way of other imaging techniques.

ENDOSCOPIC ULTRASONOGRAPHY. Endoscopic U/S (EUS) provides more detailed structural information of the pancreas compared to routine U/S and CT scan. EUS allows for evaluation of ductal and parenchymal changes, such as echotexture of the gland, calcifications, lobulations, and bands of fibrosis.

Treatment of Pain

AVOIDANCE OF ALCOHOL. Avoiding alcohol consumption decreases the frequency and severity of abdominal pain in chronic alcoholic pancreatitis. All patients with excessive alcohol consumption should be referred to an appropriate treatment program. In patients who maintain significant exocrine secretory function, pain may be provoked by alcohol, which acts as a secretagogue. In patients whose exocrine secretion is drastically reduced, alcohol plays a lesser role in the mechanism of pain. Further studies are needed to clarify the role of alcohol in pain production.

ANALGESICS. Analgesics remain the main method for pain control in chronic pancreatitis. Initially, nonnarcotic analgesics, such as salicylates or acetaminophen, should be used. As the severity of pain increases, the dose or frequency of these simpler analgesics should be increased before switching to narcotics. In severe cases, however, opiate analgesics are required.

CELIAC PLEXUS BLOCK. Celiac ganglion injection has been used for control of pancreatic pain. In small, uncontrolled series of patients with chronic pancreatitis with debilitating pain, this procedure has produced mixed results. The occasional benefits almost never last for more than a few months, and repeated treatment may not be as effective. The risks of this procedure make this an unattractive option for most patients.

ENZYME THERAPY. Several groups of investigators confirmed that intestinal administration of trypsin or chymotrypsin inhibits pancreatic enzyme secretion. It is possible that decreased enzyme secretion may result in hyperstimulation of the pancreas (secondary to elevated plasma CCK levels), resulting in pain. It has been proposed that effective enzyme replacement therapy should reduce pancreatic stimulation, decrease intraductal pressure, and diminish pain. It seems reasonable to initiate a trial of high dose, nonenteric-coated oral pancreatic enzymes (pancrelipase, 4000–33,000 U PO with meals and snacks) taken with meals for several weeks in any patient with painful chronic pancreatitis. The best results may be seen in pancreatitis of nonalcoholic etiology, with symptoms of constant, rather than recurrent, pain and only mild to moderate pancreatic insufficiency.

OCTREOTIDE. Somatostatin is a naturally occurring hormone that has been shown to inhibit pancreatic secretion. Octreotide is a synthetic long-acting analog of somatostatin that has been shown to inhibit CCK release, basal pancreatic secretion, and neural-stimulated pancreatic secretion. A randomized study of patients with advanced chronic pancreatitis and severe pain was performed. Although results did not reach statistical significance, 200 μg tid of octreotide (Sandostatin) produced the greatest pain relief (65% vs 35% of patients with placebo), especially in patients with constant as opposed to intermittent pain. Additional studies are needed to clarify the role of octreotide in the management of chronic pancreatitis pain.

ENDOSCOPIC THERAPY. Endoscopic therapy has been used for control of pain in chronic pancreatitis, with the aim of alleviating obstruction of flow caused by ductal strictures, stones, or papillary stenosis. Ductal strictures are sometimes treated by balloons or dilating catheters, but in most cases, dilation is followed by stent placement across the stricture. Endoscopic techniques also have been used for the removal of pancreatic stones in chronic pancreatitis.

SURGICAL TREATMENT. After all medical measures have failed to relieve pain, surgery should be considered. The type of surgery is selected according to the perceived mechanism for the pain, the severity of pain, ductal morphology, and the extent of parenchymal disease. Patients who have ductal dilation have a 70–80% chance of obtaining pain relief with either a partial resection with pancreaticojejunostomy or lateral pancreaticojejunostomy. Patients with moderate to severe parenchymal disease and no ductal dilation should be considered for partial pancreatic resection. Distal pancreatectomy is recommended for patients with diffuse parenchymal disease, whereas local resection of the major site of involvement may be sufficient for those with regional parenchymal disease.

Treatment of Exocrine Insufficiency

The ideal pancreatic enzyme has not been developed. Although it is not common to see complete correction of steatorrhea in patients with chronic pancreatitis, it is possible to bring the steatorrhea under control. Porcine pancreatic enzymes are the cornerstone of chronic pancreatic therapy. The clinician must be sure that the formulation is potent and will deliver lipase to the duodenum to decrease steatorrhea. It is critical that sufficient amounts of enzyme tablets be given (e.g., eight tablets of Viokase with each meal) to abolish azotorrhea and significantly reduce steatorrhea. Most patients on this regimen achieve satisfactory nutritional status and become relatively asymptomatic. In some of the symptomatic patients, the number of tablets given before meals can be increased or the amount of dietary fat reduced. These measures usually are effective in alleviating symptoms.

CYSTIC FIBROSIS

Causes

Pathophysiology

Cystic fibrosis (CF) is an autosomal-recessive disease that occurs in 1 in 2000–3000 live white births. The mutation occurs in a gene that encodes a protein called the *CF transmembrane conductance regulator*. Dysfunction of this protein results in thickened secretions in the pulmonary, intestinal, and hepatobiliary systems. Obstructive lung disease accounts for much of the morbidity and almost all of the mortality associated with CF beyond the neonatal period. GI, nutritional, and hepatobiliary complications are becoming increasingly frequent as the average age of survival increases.

More than 80% of patients with CF have pancreatic insufficiency at the time of diagnosis, and even more have partial impairment in enzyme secretion.

Presentation

Clinical Presentation

The patient's appearance can range from a severely malnourished, growth-stunted adolescent to a healthy adult. The disease should be suspected in any child with recurrent upper and lower respiratory tract symptoms. GI symptoms are usually due to pancreatic insufficiency and involve maldigestion and failure to gain weight. Patients often describe bulky, frequent, foul-smelling stools. Fat and protein maldigestion and fecal loss are the primary manifestations of pancreatic involvement of CF. Glucose intolerance is seen in 30–40% of patients with CF, but clinically significant diabetes is seen in only 3–8% of patients.

Management

Diagnostic Evaluation

- To make a diagnosis of CF, the patient must have a compatible clinical disease plus at least one of three lab findings: an abnormal sweat test, an abnormal nasal potential difference, or a genotype consisting of two CF-causing mutations.
- Duodenal aspirates from patients with CF and pancreatic insufficiency are of small volume and viscous and contain low concentrations of enzyme and bicarbonate.
- CCK or secretin fails to stimulate fluid and enzyme secretion.
- Mutations in the CF transmembrane conductance regulator have been found 11 times more frequently than expected in patients with chronic idiopathic pancreatitis.

Treatment

PANCREATIC EXTRACTS. The goal is to deliver adequate concentrations of digestive enzymes; however, fat absorption almost never returns to normal. Enteric-coated microspheres are the preferred method of delivery [pancrelipase (Creon, Pancrease)]. These enzymes require an alkaline pH to work. As CF patients have a more acidic duodenum than control subjects, the addition of acid-reducing medication may improve effectiveness. Dosages range from 500 to 2000 U of lipase activity/kg of body weight/meal. Half the dose can be given with snacks. The total dose should not exceed 10,000 lipase U/kg/day.

VITAMINS. Fat malabsorption places all CF patients at risk for fat-soluble vitamin deficiencies. Low levels of vitamins A, D, and E can be detected at 2 mos. In such patients, there may be no clinical signs, although vitamin levels may be low. Monitoring vitamin levels is an important part of management.

PANCREATIC CANCER

Approximately 28,000 new cases of pancreatic cancer occur every year in the United States, and almost all of these patients eventually die from the disease. Although surgical resection of the tumor offers the only chance for cure, even after a "curative resection," the median duration of survival is only 18–20 mos, and the 5-yr survival rate is 10%. The peak incidence of pancreatic carcinoma occurs in the seventh decade of life, and there is a slight male to female predominance. The overall incidence of the disease is 30–40% higher in the African-American population than in Caucasians. Risk factors related to pancreatic cancer are listed below.

Causes

Pathophysiology

Ductal adenocarcinoma and its variants make up >90% of all malignant exocrine pancreatic tumors. Approximately two-thirds of ductal adenocarcinomas occur in the head of the gland, with the rest in the body or tail. Tumors of the head of the pancreas are usually ≥ 2 cm in diameter, and 70–80% have metastasized to regional lymph nodes by the time they are discovered. Tumors of the body and tail commonly are more advanced and larger (5–7 cm) when they are discovered, because they do not produce symptoms as early as pancreatic head tumors. The symptoms from tumors in the body and tail are usually caused by malignant infiltration of the retroperitoneal structures, which produces pain. By the time the diagnosis is made, almost all are unresectable. The best outcome is seen in patients who have well-differentiated neoplasms, without retroperitoneal invasion or lymph node metastases. Because pancreatic cancer has usually spread to lymph nodes by the time the diagnosis is made, the majority of patients have at least stage III disease. Patients with stage IV disease (distant metastases) cannot be cured and are considered to be unresectable.

Presentation

Risk Factors
SMOKING.   Around the world, the risk factor most strongly linked to pancreatic cancer is cigarette smoking. It approximately doubles the chance of developing the disease. The risk of pancreatic cancer rapidly decreases when individuals discontinue cigarette use. The relative risk falls to approximately 1 only 10–15 yrs after quitting.

PANCREATITIS.   Epidemiologic studies suggest that the relative risk of developing pancreatic cancer in patients with chronic pancreatitis is increased by up to 15 times when compared to control populations. This suggests that changes associated with chronic inflammation and fibrosis in the pancreas are important in the development of cancer. Chronic pancreatitis, however, accounts for only a small fraction of patients who have pancreatic cancer.

SURGERY.   Patients who have undergone a partial gastrectomy have a three- to sevenfold greater risk of developing pancreatic cancer. The apparent increase in incidence may be caused by altered metabolism of ingested carcinogens by the remaining stomach and small intestine after surgery.

DIET.   Meats and foods of animal origin increase the risk of pancreatic cancer, whereas foods of plant origin and dietary fiber appear to be protective.

Clinical Presentation
PAIN.   Pain may be due to gallbladder and bile duct distention associated with biliary obstruction, pancreatic duct distention associated with pancreatic duct obstruction, or invasion of retroperitoneal or somatic nerves. Abdominal pain is most commonly felt in the epigastrium, but it also may be felt on either side or in the lower quadrants.

JAUNDICE.   Jaundice, accompanied by pain, is the presenting symptom in 80–90% of patients with cancer of the head of the pancreas.

WEIGHT LOSS.   By the time the diagnosis is made, weight loss of >10% ideal body weight is common. Pain associated with the tumor produces anorexia. The decreased food intake leads to weight loss. Malabsorption can also contribute to weight loss.

DIABETES MELLITUS.   Diabetes sometimes appears as an early manifestation of pancreatic cancer, occurring many months before the tumor becomes evident.

OTHER CLINICAL FEATURES.   Light-colored stools and dark urine are seen if there is obstructive jaundice. Other symptoms include pruritus, nausea, emesis, and weakness. Emesis may be due to duodenal or gastric outlet obstruction caused by tumor invasion. GI bleeding may occur from direct invasion of the tumor into the duodenum, stomach, or colon. There is also a poorly understood association with major depression.

Management

Diagnostic Evaluation
There are two main goals in the workup of a patient with presumed pancreatic cancer: (1) Establish the diagnosis with certainty, and (2) determine if the patient should undergo a surgical procedure to resect or palliate the disease.

CARBOHYDRATE ANTIGEN 19-9 LEVELS.   Carbohydrate antigen (CA) 19-9 is the most sensitive (80%) and specific (90%) tumor marker for pancreatic cancer. However, it is almost never positive with small tumors (<1 cm). CA 19-9 values also may be abnormal with other cancers (gastric, colorectal cancer) and with some benign conditions (cholangitis). Determination of serum CA 19-9 levels may be useful to provide some assurance that the tumor has been resected in its entirety, to signal the presence of recurrent disease after resection, and to determine the response to adjuvant therapy.

ULTRASOUND. U/S may be useful in patients with jaundice to distinguish between intrahepatic and extrahepatic causes. Extrahepatic obstruction from a pancreatic (or any periampullary) cancer is expected to show dilated intrahepatic and extrahepatic biliary ducts.

CT SCAN. Currently, helical CT is the best overall study for diagnosis as well as the preop staging of pancreatic cancer. It provides information about site of the lesion, its resectability (e.g., presence of hepatic metastases, vascular invasion), and its vascular anatomy. The primary lesion itself, as well as liver metastases, may be evident with the helical CT (which may not be seen with a standard scan). CT scan is able to detect tumors approximately ≥ 2 cm in diameter, which appear as lucent areas, because they are less well perfused with blood than the adjacent pancreatic tissue.

MRI. MRI may provide slightly better pancreatic tissue contrast than CT, but the spatial resolution is inferior.

ENDOSCOPIC RETROGRADE CHOLANGIOPANCREATOGRAPHY. ERCP has a sensitivity of 95% and a specificity of 85% for the diagnosis of pancreatic cancer. It can be performed successfully in >90% of patients, and it detects some tumors not seen on CT. At the time of ERCP, brushings for cytology may be obtained from the pancreatic duct, which has a sensitivity of approximately 60% in proving the diagnosis of malignancy. In addition, a stent also can be placed into the obstructed common bile duct, which has an important role in the palliation of patients who are not surgical candidates. In spite of its value, ERCP is not required in all patients with pancreatic cancer. If a patient has a history typical for pancreatic cancer (e.g., pain, jaundice, weight loss) with a mass in the head of the pancreas evident on CT scan, then an ERCP is unnecessary for the diagnosis and generally adds nothing to the workup that is of value to either the patient or the surgeon. If the CT scan does not show a mass or raises questions about the diagnosis, ERCP should be performed.

ENDOSCOPIC U/S. EUS is a newer technique that can provide information about whether the cancer invades adjacent vessels (which is important in making decisions about resection and whether the patient is a candidate for operation). EUS also allows fine-needle aspiration (FNA) of pancreatic lesions. It is unclear whether EUS provides more reliable information about resectability than do helical CT scans.

FINE-NEEDLE ASPIRATION. FNA for cytology can be obtained percutaneously using a fine-gauge needle under CT or U/S guidance or by EUS. FNA should not be done routinely in the workup but only when cytologic proof of malignancy alters management. For example, in a patient with an unresectable tumor in the body of the pancreas who has no symptoms for which surgical palliation is required, FNA could confirm the diagnosis, and chemotherapy, radiation, or both could be given. A patient with obstructive jaundice and a mass in the head of the pancreas may not be a candidate for resection because of coexisting medical problems. FNA could be useful to confirm the diagnosis of pancreatic cancer, and a stent could be placed to palliate the jaundice. In this manner, surgery simply to obtain tissue for diagnosis is avoided. A negative FNA never rules out the possibility of malignancy.

Treatment

SURGERY. A pancreaticoduodenectomy (Whipple resection) involves a partial gastrectomy (antrectomy), cholecystectomy, and removal of the distal common bile duct, head of the pancreas, duodenum, proximal jejunum, and regional lymph nodes. Reconstruction requires a pancreaticojejunostomy, hepaticojejunostomy, and a gastrojejunostomy. The surgery is only performed if there is no evidence of metastatic disease, and it is done for curative intent.

SURGICAL PALLIATION. When resection of the primary tumor is not possible, palliative procedures should be done. Bypass to relieve biliary obstruction is the most common procedure. An anastomosis between the gallbladder and jejunum (cholecystojejunostomy) or common bile duct and jejunum (choledochojejunostomy) are both effective bypass procedures. 15–20% of patients develop duodenal obstruction before they die. Therefore, most surgeons perform a prophylactic gastrojejunostomy at the same time as a biliary bypass. NONSURGICAL PALLIATION. Endoscopically placed metal or plastic stents can be used to relieve obstruction, thus saving patients from an operation. The stents often become occluded and need to be replaced after a certain period of time. Larger metal stents may last longer. Surgical bypass tends to stay patent longer than stents. Generally, if the life expectancy is >6 mos, surgical bypass should be considered rather than stent placement.

ADJUVANT CHEMOTHERAPY. 5-Fluorouracil, combined with radiation therapy, confers a modest prolongation of survival in patients with locally advanced pancreatic cancer. Gemcitabine has been shown to increase the quality of life in patients with advanced pancreatic cancer, but survival is only moderately improved.

KEY POINTS TO REMEMBER

- Gallstone disease and excessive alcohol use account for 70–80% of cases of acute pancreatitis in industrialized countries.
- The hallmark of acute pancreatitis is abdominal pain that is typically located in the epigastrium and periumbilical area and radiates to the back.
- Treatment of acute pancreatitis is supportive with bed rest, no oral intake, IV hydration, electrolyte replacement, and analgesia (meperidine or morphine).
- Alcohol in Western societies (70–80%) and malnutrition worldwide are the major etiologies of chronic pancreatitis.
- When exocrine secretion of pancreatic enzymes is reduced to <10%, diarrhea, steatorrhea, and azotorrhea can occur. These symptoms tend to occur relatively late in the course of chronic pancreatitis.
- Avoiding alcohol consumption decreases the frequency and severity of abdominal pain in chronic alcoholic pancreatitis.
- GI symptoms in CF are usually due to pancreatic insufficiency and involve maldigestion and inability to gain weight.
- The median duration of survival for pancreatic cancer is only 18–20 mos, and the 5-yr survival rate is 10%.
- A Whipple procedure is only performed with pancreatic cancer if there is no evidence of metastatic disease, and it is done for curative intent.

REFERENCES AND SUGGESTED READINGS

Chitkara DK, Lopez MJ, Grand RJ. Gastrointestinal complications of cystic fibrosis. *Clin Perspect Gastroenterol* 2000;3(4):201–208.

Etemad B, Whitcomb DC. Chronic pancreatitis: diagnosis, classification, and new genetic developments. *Gastroenterology* 2001;120:682–707.

Fauci AS, Braunwald E, Isselbacher KJ, et al, eds. *Harrison's principles of internal medicine*, 14th ed. New York: McGraw-Hill, 1998.

Grendall JH. Acute pancreatitis. *Clin Perspect Gastroenterol* 2000;3(6):327–333.

Mergener K, Baillie J. Acute pancreatitis. *BMJ* 1998;316:44–48.

Yamada T. *Textbook and atlas of gastroenterology on CD-ROM*. Philadelphia: Lippincott Williams & Wilkins, 1999.

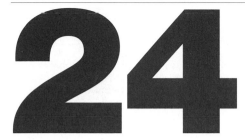

Biliary Tract Disorders

Aaron Shiels

INTRODUCTION

Diseases of the biliary tract are common disorders frequently encountered in both primary care settings and tertiary care centers. These represent a broad spectrum of diseases ranging from benign gallstone-associated conditions to primary disorders of the biliary tree to life-threatening malignancies. Because of the prevalence of biliary disease, all physicians should be familiar with the diagnosis and management of these conditions.

GALLSTONES

Cholelithiasis, the presence of stones in the gallbladder, is an extremely common disorder. The prevalence of cholelithiasis ranges from 10–15% in 40-yr-old white women to as high as 70% in female Pima Indians. Risk factors for gallstones depend on the type of stone. Cholesterol stones account for 75–90% of gallstones and are seen with increased frequency in female patients, multiparity, pregnancy, obesity, Crohn's disease, total parenteral nutrition, and Native Americans. Pigmented stones comprise the remainder and are seen more commonly with cirrhosis and chronic hemolysis, especially sickle cell disease and hereditary spherocytosis.

Causes

Natural History

Although cholelithiasis is a common condition, most patients with gallstones remain asymptomatic. Estimates of the incidence of developing a complication from gallstones are variable, but approximately 80% of patients with gallstones never develop symptoms. The incidence of developing biliary pain is approximately 1–2%/yr. In patients who develop a first episode of biliary pain, there is a 1%/yr risk of developing a severe complication. These are important figures to know, as many patients present with incidentally detected gallstones and may request recommendations regarding management.

Pathophysiology

Complications occur when gallstones occlude the cystic duct, pass into the common bile duct, or erode through the wall of the gallbladder. The common manifestations of gallstones are asymptomatic cholelithiasis, biliary pain, acute cholecystitis, choledocholithiasis, acute cholangitis, gallstone pancreatitis, and gallstone ileus. The diagnosis and management of these are discussed individually below.

Management

Diagnostic Evaluation and Treatment

ASYMPTOMATIC CHOLELITHIASIS. The diagnosis of gallstones is often made incidentally during evaluation of other conditions. U/S remains the best test for gallstones, with 95% sensitivity and 95% specificity for gallbladder stones. The yield is highest after fasting, and stones are identified by the presence of echogenic objects that produce acoustic shadowing. Gallbladder sludge may also be seen as echogenic material that layers but does not produce acoustic shadowing. Cholelithiasis may also be identified with CT scanning, although the sensitivity is lower than that of U/S. Because 80% of patients remain asymptomatic, the consensus is that prophylactic cholecystectomy is not indicated. Most patients are managed conservatively. An important exception is the patient with a calcified or "porcelain" gallbladder. Because these patients are at very high risk for gallbladder cancer, cholecystectomy should be performed in the absence of symptoms.

BILIARY PAIN. The term classically used to describe the condition of biliary pain is biliary colic, but this is a misnomer because the pain is not usually colicky. Patients with biliary pain describe episodes of epigastric or right upper quadrant pain that may radiate to the right scapula or shoulder. The pain gradually increases over 30 mins and then plateaus for ≥ 1 hr before subsiding. There may be associated dyspeptic symptoms, including bloating, nausea, or vomiting. The interval between attacks is variable, and weeks or months may pass between episodes. The pain is caused by transient occlusion of the cystic duct neck by a gallstone. Diagnosis of biliary pain requires the appropriate clinical presentation in the setting of documented cholelithiasis. At first glance, this appears to be a fairly simple diagnosis. However, because gallstones are so common, many patients present with atypical pain or dyspepsia and cholelithiasis. Clinical judgment is required to determine whether symptoms are related to gallstones. Laparoscopic cholecystectomy is the treatment of choice, but open cholecystectomy is required in a minority of patients. In one study, 88% of patients had relief of symptoms after cholecystectomy. For patients who are poor surgical candidates, oral dissolution therapy with ursodiol or chenodiol may be used, but only 20–30% have dissolution of stones.

ACUTE CHOLECYSTITIS. Gallstones account for 95% of cases of acute cholecystitis. The remainder are termed *acalculous cholecystitis* and are seen in the critically ill. Cystic duct occlusion results in bile stasis, gallbladder wall edema, gallbladder distention, and inflammatory exudate. Patients typically present with steady upper abdominal pain that lasts >4 hrs. It may be difficult to distinguish the pain of acute cholecystitis from prolonged biliary pain. Associated nausea, vomiting, and fever may be present. The presentation may be more subtle in the elderly. If bacteremic, patients may present with a more toxic presentation, including high fever, rigors, and severe abdominal tenderness. Exam often reveals right upper quadrant tenderness or a positive Murphy's sign (pain with palpation of the right upper quadrant during inspiration). Most patients have a modest leukocytosis and normal or only slightly increased transaminases, bilirubin, and lipase. Significantly increased transaminases or lipase should raise suspicion of a common duct stone. Patients with suspected acute cholecystitis should undergo U/S. Important findings include gallstones, sonographic Murphy's sign, gallbladder wall thickening, and pericholecystic fluid. If the diagnosis remains in doubt, cholescintigraphy (hepatoiminodiacetic acid, paraisopropyliminodiacetic acid, or diisopropyl iminodiacetic acid scan) should be performed. In this study, patients are given radio-labeled iminodiacetic acid derivatives. These are rapidly extracted by the liver and then excreted into bile. A normal study shows radioactivity in the gallbladder, common bile duct, and small intestine within 60 mins. In acute cholecystitis, there is nonfilling of the gallbladder due to cystic duct obstruction. Patients with acute cholecystitis are made NPO and given IV fluids and broad-spectrum antibiotics. NG suction is performed if the patient is distended or vomiting. Prompt surgical consultation should be obtained. Definitive management is laparoscopic or open cholecystectomy. Most clinicians recommend waiting 24–48 hrs until the patient has stabilized, but surgery should be performed more urgently if the condition deteriorates. Patients who are poor surgical candidates should undergo percutaneous cholecystostomy. Complications of acute cholecystitis include gallbladder perforation, emphysematous cholecystitis due to gas-forming bacteria, and gallstone ileus (see below).

CHOLEDOCHOLITHIASIS. Stones may pass from the gallbladder into the common bile duct or form de novo in the bile ducts. Retained common bile duct stones may be present for years after cholecystectomy before causing any problems. The stones commonly become impacted at the ampulla of Vater. Patients may be asymptomatic or present with a broad range of syndromes, including biliary pain, jaundice, cholangitis, or pancreatitis. Usual lab abnormalities include increased transaminases, alkaline phosphatase, bilirubin, amylase, and lipase. The best initial diagnostic study is U/S, which is very sensitive for cholelithiasis and dilated bile ducts but less sensitive (30–50%) for common bile duct stones. An important point is that the *absence of ductal dilatation does not exclude choledocholithiasis*. CT scanning may also be useful but also has lower sensitivity for common bile duct stones. If U/S demonstrates dilated ducts or choledocholithiasis, or if suspicion of a common duct stone remains despite an equivocal U/S, then endoscopic retrograde cholangiopancreatography (ERCP) should be performed. ERCP is very accurate for diagnosing stones and allows definitive treatment with sphincterotomy and stone extraction. Patients who have common duct stones identified during laparoscopic cholecystectomy should have either intraoperative duct exploration or postoperative ERCP with sphincterotomy and stone extraction.

ACUTE CHOLANGITIS. Choledocholithiasis causes most cases of cholangitis, with neoplasms and biliary strictures accounting for the other cases. Cholangitis occurs when bacterial infection complicates an obstructed duct. Approximately 70% of patients present with all three components of Charcot's triad: pain, jaundice, and fever. If suppurative cholangitis develops, patients will present with mental status changes and hypotension. Leukocytosis and increased bilirubin and alkaline phosphatase are usually present. Blood cultures are frequently positive, especially with suppurative cholangitis. The most common organisms isolated are gram-negative rods, enterococci, and anaerobes. Broad-spectrum antibiotics should be started if cholangitis is suspected. The diagnosis must then be made quickly, as patients are at risk of developing severe sepsis. U/S or abdominal CT should be performed, looking for ductal dilatation or common bile duct stones. However, a negative study does not rule out cholangitis, as the common duct may not be dilated early in the course of disease, and common duct stones may be missed. ERCP is the procedure of choice for suspected cases of cholangitis. ERCP identifies common duct stones or strictures and allows therapeutic interventions with sphincterotomy, biliary drainage, stone extraction, and biliary stent placement. If ERCP is unsuccessful or cannot be performed, then percutaneous transhepatic cholangiography (PTC) or surgical decompression should be pursued.

GALLSTONE PANCREATITIS. Gallstone pancreatitis is discussed in detail in Chap. 23, Pancreatic Disorders.

GALLSTONE ILEUS. Gallstones may erode through the wall of the gallbladder into the small intestine. The stones then may cause obstruction at any bowel segment, but the terminal ileum is the most common location. Patients present with symptoms and exam findings consistent with bowel obstruction. The diagnosis is suggested by the findings of air in the biliary tree with dilated loops of bowel and air fluid levels on x-ray. Treatment is surgical with closure of the cholecystenteric fistula and enterotomy with removal of the stones.

PRIMARY SCLEROSING CHOLANGITIS

Primary sclerosing cholangitis (PSC) is a chronic cholestatic liver disease that affects both the intrahepatic and extrahepatic bile ducts. 75% of patients are male, and the average age at diagnosis is 40 yrs. Up to 70% of PSC occurs in the setting of inflammatory bowel disease (IBD), with ulcerative colitis accounting for 90% of those cases. There is no relation between the duration and severity of IBD and the development of PSC. Although colectomy is curative for ulcerative colitis, it does not eliminate the risk of PSC.

Causes

Pathophysiology
The etiology of PSC is unknown. Both intrahepatic and extrahepatic bile ducts are involved with strictures. The disease process is usually diffuse, with strictures distributed throughout the biliary system. Strictures, especially large strictures, predispose the

patient to intermittent obstruction to biliary flow with subsequent bacterial cholangitis. Obstruction of biliary flow causes reflux of bile into the hepatocytes. Pruritus due to deposition of bile acids in the skin can be severe. Steatorrhea and malabsorption of fat-soluble vitamins may develop late in disease due to decreased secretion of bile acids. Metabolic bone disease, most commonly osteoporosis, occurs frequently in PSC for unclear reasons.

Management

Diagnostic Evaluation
The onset of disease is often insidious with the gradual onset of fatigue, pruritus, and jaundice. If advanced liver disease has already developed, some patients present with variceal bleeding, encephalopathy, or ascites. A substantial number of patients are diagnosed based on abnormal lab tests before symptoms have started. Most have significantly elevated alkaline phosphatase, gamma-glutamyltransferase, and bilirubin. The transaminases are elevated to a lesser degree. Patients with IBD who present with **increased alkaline phosphatase** should have an aggressive evaluation for PSC. Definitive diagnosis is made by imaging of the biliary tree with either ERCP or PTC. Magnetic resonance cholangiopancreatography may also help make diagnosis. The classic finding is multifocal stricturing of the intrahepatic and extrahepatic bile ducts with intervening normal or dilated segments. This is often described as a "*string of beads*." A minority of patients do not have the classic cholangiographic findings but do have small duct cholangitis identified on liver biopsy.

Treatment
PSC follows a slowly progressive course, with a median survival of approximately 10 yrs from the time of diagnosis. Medical therapy has not proved successful in slowing progression of disease. Management is therefore primarily supportive until end-stage liver disease (ESLD) develops, at which time liver transplantation is offered. Indications for transplantation include refractory ascites, recurrent bacterial cholangitis, encephalopathy, and variceal bleeding. The specific complications are managed as follows.
    PRURITUS. Pruritus can be particularly severe in PSC and can be difficult to manage. Symptoms often respond to bile acid–binding resins, such as cholestyramine, 4 g PO bid–qid. Other options include ursodiol, ultraviolet phototherapy, antihistamines, or phenobarbital.
    BACTERIAL CHOLANGITIS. Bacterial cholangitis more commonly occurs in patients who have had manipulation of the biliary tract or have developed a dominant stricture. Cholelithiasis or choledocholithiasis may also contribute to the development of bacterial cholangitis. Patients present with fever and worsening jaundice and may have recurring episodes. Treatment is directed at relieving the obstruction, usually endoscopically. ERCP allows stenting of large strictures, biliary decompression, and removal of stones. Long-term prophylactic antibiotics may be used in recurrent cholangitis.
    DOMINANT STRICTURE. Approximately 20% develop a dominant stricture, presenting with fever, pruritus, and jaundice. Cholangiography demonstrates the dominant stricture and balloon dilatation can be performed on benign strictures. However, it is often very difficult to differentiate a dominant stricture from cholangiocarcinoma. Tumor markers such as carbohydrate antigen 19-9 and carcinoembryonic antigen (CEA) may be of some value in identifying patients with cholangiocarcinoma.
    CHOLANGIOCARCINOMA. Patients with PSC have a 10–30% chance of developing bile duct cancer. This is often very difficult to diagnose in the setting of PSC. The management of cholangiocarcinoma is discussed below.
    PORTAL HYPERTENSION. Advanced PSC eventually leads to ESLD with the subsequent development of portal HTN. Variceal bleeding, portosystemic encephalopathy, and ascites are managed as with other types of ESLD. Liver transplantation is the treatment of choice in patients with ESLD from PSC.

CHOLANGIOCARCINOMA

Bile duct cancer is a relatively rare tumor seen primarily in middle-aged men. The strongest association is seen with PSC, but it is also associated with cystic biliary disease, ulcerative colitis, and chronic liver fluke infestation. Patients typically present with anorexia, weight loss, abdominal pain, pruritus, and jaundice. A Klatskin's tumor is a bile duct cancer with involvement of the hilum of the right and left hepatic ducts. Some bile duct tumors spread diffusely throughout the liver, making it difficult to distinguish from PSC. Most tumors are locally invasive and do not usually metastasize.

Management

Diagnostic Evaluation
Most patients have increased alkaline phosphatase and bilirubin. U/S and abdominal CT scanning are useful in identifying intrahepatic or extrahepatic ductal dilation, but the primary tumors are often difficult to visualize. MRI or magnetic resonance cholangiopancreatography may be more sensitive in identifying the primary tumor. ERCP or PTC provides direct imaging of biliary system and can define the extent of tumor spread. Tissue diagnosis can be made using bile cytology, cytologic brushings, cholangioscopic biopsies, or percutaneous fine-needle aspiration. The histologic diagnosis of cholangiocarcinoma may be challenging, as many tumors are well differentiated and occur in the setting of PSC. Carbohydrate antigen 19-9 and CEA are tumor markers that may assist in differentiating cholangiocarcinoma from PSC.

Treatment
Surgical resection represents the only option for long-term survival. Distal duct tumors are more likely to be resectable than proximal tumors. Median survival for resectable tumors is 3 yrs but only 1 yr if unresectable. Patients who have unresectable tumors may be candidates for palliative biliary-enteric anastomosis or biliary stenting by ERCP. Radiation may be used as a palliative treatment. Bile duct cancers respond poorly to chemotherapy. Death usually results from recurrent biliary sepsis or liver abscess formation.

GALLBLADDER CARCINOMA

Gallbladder cancer represents the most common biliary tract malignancy. It is a disease predominantly seen in elderly women. Up to 80% have a history of gallstones, and there is a higher incidence with longer duration of gallstones. It is the most common GI malignancy in Native Americans. Patients who have a calcified or "porcelain" gallbladder are at very high risk of gallbladder cancer and should undergo cholecystectomy even if asymptomatic. Patients typically present with abdominal pain, which may be difficult to differentiate from biliary pain, or acute cholecystitis. Other common symptoms include nausea, vomiting, weight loss, and jaundice.

Management

Diagnostic Evaluation
U/S often detects masses within the gallbladder lumen, gallbladder wall thickening, or gallstones. However, a normal U/S does not rule out gallbladder cancer. CT scanning demonstrates masses and gallbladder thickening and provides additional evidence for extent of disease. ERCP or PTC is indicated in patients with evidence of biliary obstruction. Cholangiography may also permit stent placement for biliary decompression. Histologic diagnosis in tumors that appear unresectable can be accomplished by percutaneous biopsy. If resection is planned, then preop tissue diagnosis is unnecessary.

Treatment
Most patients present with advanced unresectable disease. The overall 5-yr survival rate is <5%. Patients with unresectable disease may receive chemotherapy or palliative treatment with endoscopic stent placement. Approximately 15–30% of patients have potentially resectable tumors. Depending on the extent of spread, surgery may be as simple as cholecystectomy or require extensive hepatic, pancreatic, and duodenal resection.

KEY POINTS TO REMEMBER

* Eighty percent of patients with gallstones remain free of symptoms; therefore, prophylactic surgery is not indicated in asymptomatic cholelithiasis.
* The incidence of developing biliary pain is approximately 1–2%/yr. In patients who develop a first episode of biliary pain, there is a 1%/yr risk of developing a severe complication.
* U/S is the best test for gallstones, with 95% sensitivity and 95% specificity for gallbladder stones.
* Laparoscopic cholecystectomy is the treatment of choice for biliary pain (commonly referred to as biliary colic) in the presence of gallstones.
* U/S should be performed as the first test for suspected choledocholithiasis, but a negative study does not rule out common bile duct stones. ERCP is the definitive diagnostic and therapeutic procedure for suspected choledocholithiasis.
* PSC is best diagnosed with direct cholangiography (ERCP or PTC), which demonstrates "string of beads." Magnetic resonance cholangiopancreatography is a useful alternative.
* Up to 70% of cases of PSC occur in patients with IBD (ulcerative colitis much more commonly than Crohn's).
* Prophylactic cholecystectomy should be performed in patients with a calcified or "porcelain" gallbladder because of the increased risk of gallbladder cancer.

REFERENCES AND SUGGESTED READINGS

Diehl AK. Epidemiology and natural history of gallstone disease. *Gastroenterol Clin North Am* 1991;20:1–19.

Freeman ML, Nelson DB, Sherman S. Complications of endoscopic biliary sphincterotomy. *N Engl J Med* 1996;335:909–918.

Jones RS. Carcinoma of the gallbladder. *Surg Clin North Am* 1990;70:1419–1428.

Kadakia SC. Biliary tract emergencies: acute cholecystitis, acute cholangitis and acute pancreatitis. *Med Clin North Am* 1993;77:1015–1036.

Lai ECS, Mok FPT, Tan ESY. Endoscopic biliary drainage for severe acute cholangitis. *N Engl J Med* 1992;326:1582–1586.

Lee YM, Kaplan MM. Primary sclerosing cholangitis. *N Engl J Med* 1995;332:924–937.

Rosen CB, Nagorney DM, Wiesner RH. Cholangiocarcinoma complicating primary sclerosing cholangitis. *Ann Surg* 1991;213:21–25.

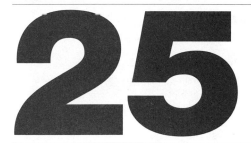

Gastrointestinal Procedures

David S. Lotsoff

INTRODUCTION

The ability to perform endoscopic procedures has radically changed the practice of gastroenterology. **Endoscopy** allows for direct visual inspection, tissue sampling, and minimally invasive therapeutic intervention. An endoscopic procedure is considered worth performing if the benefit for the patient exceeds the risks by a sufficiently wide margin. Preparation for endoscopy involves addressing important issues specific to each patient, such as assessing contraindications and relative contraindications, medication allergies, patient medications, and possible interactions with medicines used for sedation. In addition, the presence of coagulopathy, comorbid factors, and conditions potentially requiring antibiotic prophylaxis must be considered. Furthermore, each patient, or a designated guardian, should understand the benefits and risks associated with the procedure, and informed consent must be obtained before the initiation of the procedure. General indications for endoscopic procedures are listed in Table 25-1.

UPPER GASTROINTESTINAL ENDOSCOPY

Esophagogastroduodenoscopy allows high-resolution visual inspection of the upper GI tract from the esophagus to the second portion of the duodenum. At most institutions, exams are performed using topical anesthetics applied to the oropharynx in combination with IV conscious sedation. Esophagogastroduodenoscopy can be used for a variety of indications, such as the diagnosis and management of abdominal pain or upper GI bleeding, the screening and diagnosis of esophageal or gastric malignancies, and the palliation of dysphagia resulting from both malignant and benign causes. Various instruments may be passed through the therapeutic channel of the endoscope for use in tissue biopsy, medication delivery, or cauterization for the goal of hemostasis. The only patient preparation required is to avoid oral intake for ≥ 6 hrs before the procedure.

Endoscopy has a small but definite risk of complications. Significant bleeding has been reported in 0.025–0.06%. Perforation has been reported in 0.008–0.04%, and cardiorespiratory complications, mostly attributed to premedication or sedation, can occur in 0.05–0.73% of patients. The risk of mortality as a result of upper endoscopy has been estimated to range from 0.005% to 0.04%.

COLONOSCOPY

Colonoscopy can be used to visually inspect the entire colon as well as the terminal ileum. As with esophagogastroduodenoscopy, colonoscopy almost always involves the use of IV conscious sedation. Colonoscopy is performed for a variety of indications, including evaluation and treatment of overt lower GI bleeding, evaluation of iron-deficiency anemia, screening for colon cancer, diagnosis and cancer surveillance in inflammatory bowel disease, palliative treatment of stenosing or bleeding neoplasms, and evaluation of clinically significant diarrhea of unexplained origin. Various instruments may be passed through the therapeutic channel of the endoscope for use in tissue biopsy, medication delivery to the colonic mucosa, cauterization or fulguration of tissue,

TABLE 25-1.   GENERAL INDICATIONS FOR ENDOSCOPIC PROCEDURES

GI endoscopy is generally indicated

If a change in management is probable based on results of endoscopy

After an empiric trial of therapy for a suspected benign digestive disorder has been unsuccessful

As the initial method of evaluation as an alternative to radiographic studies

When a primary therapeutic procedure is contemplated

GI endoscopy is generally not indicated

When the results do not contribute to a management choice

For periodic follow-up of healed benign disease unless surveillance of a premalignant condition is warranted

GI endoscopy is generally contraindicated

When the risks to patient health or life are judged to outweigh the most favorable benefits of the procedure

When adequate patient cooperation or consent cannot be obtained

When a perforated viscus is known or suspected

---

and removal of polyps. Colon preparation is required before the procedure. This usually involves a lavage or purgative method used on the day or evening before the patient's colonoscopy. Acceptable regimens include polyethylene glycol (GoLYTELY) or Phosphosoda preparations.

Colonoscopy also has a small but definite risk of complications. Bleeding can be seen in up to 1.6% of patients, and perforation can occur in up to 0.5% of patients. Surgical consultation should be obtained in the event of suspected perforation. Cardiorespiratory complications are also a concern and are mostly attributed to the sedation used during the procedure. Mortality has been reported in up to 0.06% of patients.

FLEXIBLE SIGMOIDOSCOPY

Flexible sigmoidoscopy involves a shorter endoscope compared with colonoscopy and is used to examine the distal colon up to the splenic flexure. This exam is usually performed without sedation, which adds the advantages of decreased cost, fewer complications associated with sedation, and decreased lost work time for the patient. However, the procedure is more uncomfortable for the patient, as no sedation is given. This procedure also eliminates the need for a complete colon preparation. Two enemas given a few hours before the procedure are usually adequate preparation. The risk of perforation during flexible sigmoidoscopy is very low (0.01%). Flexible sigmoidoscopy is generally used for evaluation of suspected distal colonic disease when colonoscopy is not indicated, anastomotic recurrence in rectosigmoid carcinoma, and colon cancer screening, usually in conjunction with a barium enema.

SMALL BOWEL ENTEROSCOPY

Because standard upper GI endoscopy is limited to the level of the second portion of the duodenum, a special endoscope is needed to examine the upper GI tract beyond the ligament of Treitz. Two types of enteroscopes developed for this purpose are the Sonde enteroscope and the push enteroscope.

Sonde enteroscopes are 400 cm long and are placed into the upper GI tract and allowed to advance into the distal small bowel by peristalsis. Visualization of the intestinal mucosa is then achieved on withdrawal of the enteroscope. The procedure is limited in that only minimal therapeutic intervention is possible, and the endoscope can not be readvanced. This procedure is rarely performed.

Push enteroscopes are 160–240 cm in length and can be used for therapeutic intervention. They allow for controlled insertion and withdrawal. Push enteroscopy is traditionally used after a negative upper endoscopy and colonoscopy. The yield of push enteroscopy in this setting is approximately 60%.

Recently, a new innovation has been developed to allow visualization of the distal small bowel. Capsule enteroscopy is currently being investigated in many settings as a means to visualize segments of the bowel previously inaccessible to endoscopy. For this study, the patient swallows a capsule that contains a camera, light source, battery, and radiotransmitter. As the capsule traverses the GI tract, it takes pictures and transmits these images to a receiver that the patient wears on the belt. The capsule takes 8 hrs of images, usually enough time to traverse the ileocecal valve. The images are then loaded onto a computer where they can be viewed in a movie format at up to 25 frames/sec. The current indications for capsule endoscopy include evaluation of obscure GI bleeding and persistent occult GI bleeding. The major contraindication is the presence of intestinal strictures, as this would prevent passage of the capsule. The exact role of this study has yet to be fully determined.

ENDOSCOPIC RETROGRADE CHOLANGIOPANCREATOGRAPHY

Endoscopic retrograde cholangiopancreatography (ERCP) is performed using a specially designed endoscope that involves a side-viewing imaging system. This system allows direct visualization of the major and minor papillae and facilitates insertion of devices into the desired duct.

ERCP can be used effectively in detecting and treating choledocholithiasis. Sphincterotomy may be performed at the time of stone removal to reduce the chance of recurrent choledocholithiasis. ERCP may also be used therapeutically to dilate benign and malignant strictures in the biliary tree with or without subsequent stent placement. Brushings for cytology may also be obtained during ERCP to assist in the diagnosis of cholangiocarcinoma and pancreatic neoplasms.

ERCP is associated with all the risks of upper endoscopy. Approximately 5% of patients develop postprocedural pancreatitis. The incidence is higher when sphincter of Oddi manometry is performed. This is usually mild and self-limited; however, in a small percentage of cases, this can be life-threatening.

ENDOSCOPIC ULTRASONOGRAPHY

Endoscopic ultrasound (EUS) allows for high-resolution imaging of the luminal GI tract. It uses higher frequencies than transabdominal ultrasound and provides resolution of the GI tract wall into nine distinct layers that correlate closely with histology. This is of great value in the preoperative staging of GI malignancies and the evaluation of intramural and submucosal masses. In addition, diagnostic tissue sampling can be performed under EUS guidance. Specific roles for EUS include the staging of esophageal cancer (including the use of fine-needle aspiration to detect malignant lymphadenopathy), diagnosis of submucosal tumors, staging of pancreatic cancer, detection of small pancreatic and ampullary tumors, and even the staging of certain lung cancers.

LIVER BIOPSY

In some instances, histologic exam of liver tissue is necessary. Common indications for liver biopsy include evaluation of abnormal liver chemistries, assessment of degree of inflammation and fibrosis in chronic liver disease (e.g., hepatitis C), and diagnosis of liver masses. Liver biopsy may be accomplished by several different techniques. Bedside percutaneous liver biopsy is commonly performed by gastroenterologists or hepatologists. The patient is placed supine with the right arm behind the head. With U/S guidance or percussion, an appropriate biopsy location is chosen in the right lateral chest wall, usually near the eighth intercostal space. The area is sterile prepped and draped, and lidocaine is used to infiltrate the skin, subcutaneous fat, intercostal muscles, and liver capsule. A small incision is made, and the liver biopsy needle is advanced to the liver capsule. With the patient held in full expiration, the biopsy needle is advanced into the liver parenchyma, and a core of tissue is obtained. The patient is then observed closely for at least 4 hrs for complications. Contraindications to percutaneous liver biopsy include severe coagulopathy, thrombocytopenia, or ascites. If percutaneous liver biopsy cannot be safely performed, or if portal pressure measurements are needed, transjugular liver biopsy under radiologic guidance may be performed. Directed biopsy with U/S or CT guidance may be necessary for sampling of liver masses. Complications of liver biopsy are rare but can be severe. The most common complication is pain at the biopsy site or in the right shoulder. Less common complications are bleeding, pneumothorax, gallbladder perforation, inadvertent kidney biopsy, or death. Most complications are apparent within the first 4–6 hrs, but they may occur up to 48 hrs after biopsy.

CONSCIOUS SEDATION

Conscious sedation provides adequate analgesia and sedation for most GI procedures while allowing the patient to cooperate with verbal commands. Conscious sedation for endoscopic procedures usually involves a benzodiazepine (i.e., midazolam) and an opiate (i.e., meperidine). Droperidol should no longer be used as an adjunct to these medications due to the risk of cardiac arrhythmias. Propofol is a short-acting sedative, and its use requires the presence of an anesthesiologist for both the administration of the drug and airway control.

The American Society of Anesthesiology (ASA) assessment (categories I–V) is useful in evaluating the sedation risk for a patient. ASA category I represents the least risk. Advanced age, obesity, pregnancy, sleep apnea, a history of substance abuse, or severe cardiac, respiratory, hepatic, renal, or CNS disease place patients at higher risk for sedation. Patients should be made NPO before their procedure to reduce the risk associated with anesthesia.

The most common sedation complications include airway obstruction and respiratory depression, oversedation, hypoxia, and hypotension. Patients are monitored during the procedure using continuous pulse oximetry, heart monitoring, and intermittent BP recordings.

ANTIBIOTIC PROPHYLAXIS FOR ENDOCARDITIS

Bacterial endocarditis is a potentially life-threatening infection. Approximately 4% of patients develop bacteremia associated with endoscopy, but this varies depending on the specific procedure performed. Prosthetic heart valves, a history of endocarditis, and surgically constructed systemic pulmonary shunts are considered higher-risk cardiac conditions. The American Society of Gastrointestinal Endoscopy guidelines regarding recommendations for the use of prophylactic antibiotics in endoscopic procedures are listed in Table 25-2.

Antibiotics should be administered 30 mins before the procedure. For upper endoscopy and/or stricture dilation, give ampicillin, 2 g IV. For all other procedures, give ampicillin, 2 g IV, plus gentamicin, 1.5 mg/kg (up to 80 mg) IV. Vancomycin, 1 g IV, is substituted for the penicillin-allergic patient. An IV cephalosporin or its equivalent should be administered to patients undergoing percutaneous endoscopic feeding tube placement.

ANTICOAGULATION AND ANTIPLATELET AGENTS

Patients who require chronic anticoagulation or antiplatelet agents pose a challenging problem when a GI procedure is needed. The bleeding risk for GI procedures is increased in the setting of anticoagulation or antiplatelet drugs, especially if polypectomy or biopsy is performed. If possible, warfarin should be discontinued ≥ 5 days before the procedure, and the INR should be checked on the day of the procedure. The

TABLE 25-2. AMERICAN SOCIETY OF GASTROINTESTINAL ENDOSCOPY RECOMMENDATIONS FOR ANTIBIOTIC PROPHYLAXIS

Antibiotics definitely recommended

    High-risk procedure (stricture dilation, varix sclerosis, ERCP) in high-risk conditions (prosthetic valve, previous endocarditis, synthetic vascular graft <1 yr old, systemic pulmonary shunt)

    Endoscopic feeding tube placement

    ERCP for obstructed bile duct or pancreatic pseudocyst

Insufficient data to make firm recommendation

    Low-risk procedure (colonoscopy, esophagogastroduodenoscopy, varix ligation) in high-risk conditions

    High-risk procedure in intermediate-risk conditions (rheumatic disease, mitral valve prolapse with regurgitation, hypertrophic cardiomyopathy, congenital heart disease)

Antibiotics not recommended

    Low-risk procedure in intermediate-risk conditions

    Any endoscopic procedure in low-risk cardiac conditions (coronary artery bypass grafting, pacemaker, automatic implantable cardioverter-defibrillator)

    Any endoscopic procedure in patients with prosthetic joints

threshold for an acceptable INR is not well established, but most endoscopists prefer the INR to be <1.5. If anticoagulation cannot be stopped for an extended period of time (mechanical valves, atrial fibrillation with known left atrial thrombus), then the patient should be admitted for conversion from warfarin to heparin. Once the INR has decreased to an acceptable level, the procedure can be safely performed by stopping heparin 6 hrs before the procedure. The timing for resuming anticoagulation depends largely on what type of procedure is performed. Aspirin and other antiplatelet agents should be discontinued ≥ 1 wk before the procedure. These recommendations are easier to follow for elective procedures. For patients with acute bleeding who require endoscopic therapy, attempts should be made to correct any coagulopathy using a combination of FFP, vitamin K, and platelets.

KEY POINTS TO REMEMBER

- EGD allows visual inspection, sampling, and treatment of lesions in the upper GI tract from the esophagus to the second portion of the duodenum.
- Colonoscopy can be used to inspect and perform interventions in the entire colon and terminal ileum.
- Capsule endoscopy is a new innovation that allows visualization of the entire small intestine.
- ERCP uses a side-viewing endoscope to examine the major and minor papilla and facilitates insertion of devices into the biliary or pancreatic ducts.
- Conscious sedation provides adequate analgesia and sedation for most GI procedures.
- Antibiotic prophylaxis is recommended for patients undergoing high-risk procedures with high-risk conditions for bacterial endocarditis.

REFERENCES AND SUGGESTED READINGS

Arrowsmith JB, Gerstman BB, Fleischer DE, et al. Results from the American Society for Gastrointestinal Endoscopy/US Food and Drug Administration collaborative study on complication rates and drug use during gastrointestinal endoscopy. *Gastrointest Endosc* 1991;37:421–427.

Berner JS, Mauer K, Lewis BS. Push and sonde enteroscopy for the diagnosis of obscure gastrointestinal bleeding. *Am J Gastroenterol* 1994;89:2139–2142.

Carlsson U, Grattidge P. Sedation for upper gastrointestinal endoscopy: a comparative study of propofol and midazolam. *Endoscopy* 1995;3:240–243.

Chong J, Tagle M, Barkin JS, et al. Small bowel push type enteroscopy for patients with occult gastrointestinal bleeding of suspected small bowel pathology. *Am J Gastroenterol* 1994;89:2143–2146.

Froehlich F, Gonvers JJ, Vader JP, et al. Appropriateness of gastrointestinal endoscopy: risk of complications. *Endoscopy* 1999;31(8):684–686.

Groveman HD, Sanowski RA, Klauber MR. Training primary care physicians in flexible sigmoidoscopy—performance evaluation of 12,167 procedures. *West J Med* 1988; 148:221–224.

Mallery S, Van Dam J. Advances in diagnostic and therapeutic endoscopy. *Med Clin North Am* 2000;84(5):1059–1083.

Index

Page numbers followed by *t* indicate tables; numbers followed by *f* indicate figures.